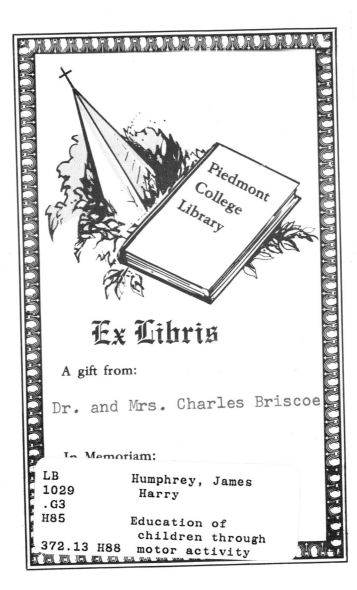

EDUCATION OF CHILDREN
THROUGH MOTOR ACTIVITY

EDUCATION OF CHILDREN THROUGH MOTOR ACTIVITY

By

JAMES H. HUMPHREY

Professor and Motor Activity Learning Specialist
University of Maryland
College Park, Maryland

With a Foreword by

Henry L. Sublett

Professor and Chairman
Department of Early Childhood-Elementary Education
University of Maryland
College Park, Maryland

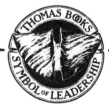

CHARLES C THOMAS • **PUBLISHER**
Springfield • *Illinois* • *U.S.A.*

Published and Distributed Throughout the World by
CHARLES C THOMAS ● PUBLISHER
Bannerstone House
301-327 East Lawrence Avenue, Springfield, Illinois, U.S.A.

© *1975, by* CHARLES C THOMAS ● PUBLISHER
ISBN 0-398-03356-0
Library of Congress Catalog Card Number: 74-26518

Printed in the United States of America
R-1

Library of Congress Cataloging in Publication Data

Humphrey, James Harry, 1911-
    Health teaching in elementary schools.

    Includes index.
    1. Health education (Elementary)   I. Johnson,
Warren Russell, 1921-   joint author.   II. Nowack,
Dorothy R., joint author.   III. Title.
LB1587.A3H85   372.3'7   74-26518
ISBN 0-398-03356-0

FOREWORD

FROM the beginning, too many writers of books for the teaching profession have seemed to feel that the quality of the book is directly related to the quantity of *theory* presented in its pages. No one would question the value of presenting the undergirding theory, but balancing attention to the matter of its implementation continues to be a need. The author of EDUCATION OF CHILDREN THROUGH MOTOR ACTIVITY has provided both, and he is to be commended for it.

In his introductory chapters, the author gives useful background material regarding learning through motor activity. He contends that the potential here has often been ignored in planning instructional experiences and cites the resulting lack of agreement with the basic laws of child growth and development. There is probably little disagreement on the matter of involving the child directly in learning activities — *learning by doing* has long been a basic tenet in planning for teaching. Actually following through on this has been slower, however. The author offers real help in this area. He treats each area of the curriculum, presenting a rationale for motor activity as an important contributor, then suggests specific learning activities to carry out the rationale. It is a *fail proof* type of help, and teachers will no doubt welcome the numerous ideas and suggestions offered here as valuable aides to their planning.

Professor Humphrey writes from a broad background of research in the field of motor activity and from a longstanding personal interest in the area. His earlier books and research reports attest to this. This new book broadens and deepens the concept of motor activity learning in general and offers provocative reading as well as practical help to educators.

Henry L. Sublett

PREFACE

CHILD learning through motor activity has received a great deal of recognition in recent years, and increasing attention of educators is being directed to this social psychological phenomenon. The use of motor activity as a medium for learning is not only supported by respectable theoretical postulation, but is backed up by sophisticated research as well. EDUCATION OF CHILDREN THROUGH MOTOR ACTIVITY has been developed with this basic premise in mind.

The introductory chapter is intended to give a general overview of the approach. Chapter Two takes into account factors which facilitate learning through motor activity, while Chapter Three considers research in this area. Chapter Four is concerned with the value of the approach for slow learning children. Chapters Five through Nine deal in some detail with how motor activities can be used specifically in such elementary school curriculum areas as reading, mathematics, science, social studies and health and safety.

The book should have a variety of uses. It could serve as a supplementary textbook in the subject areas discussed in Chapters Five through Nine. It could be helpful in teacher preparation courses in special education as well as courses concerned with learning theory and principles of learning. It should be a valuable handbook of learning activities for classroom teachers. And finally, it should be useful for parents in assisting their children with learning in the out-of-school situation.

Since the materials in the book comprise some twenty-five years of experimentation and research on the part of the author, it is impossible to acknowledge personally all of those individuals who have made a contribution to the work. The materials have undergone extensive field trials in various types of situations, and the author is most grateful to the literally thousands of children and teachers who took part in these endeavors. Special acknowledgment is due to certain staff members of the College of Education at the University of Maryland who have collaborated with the author in various projects. These include, Dr. Robert M. Wilson, Professor and Director of the Reading Center; Dr. Dorothy D. Sullivan, Professor and Reading Specialist; and Dr. Robert Ashlock, Professor and Director of the Arithmetic Center. Grateful acknowledgment is also expressed to Dr. Henry L. Sublett who analyzed the material from the point of view of the specialist in elementary education and prepared the Foreword.

J.H.H.

CONTENTS

EDUCATION OF CHILDREN THROUGH MOTOR ACTIVITY

CHAPTER ONE.

INTRODUCTION

It seems not only appropriate but imperative at the outset of this volume to present a working description of certain terminology. This is particularly true of the meaning of the approach to learning with which we are concerned — that of *motor activity.*

The term *motor,* as far as human motion is concerned, pertains to a muscle, nerve or center that effects or produces movement. That is, a nerve connecting with a muscle causes the impulse for motion known as motor impulse. The term *activity* derives from the word *active,* one meaning of which is the requirement of action. Thus, when the two words motor and activity are used together, muscular action is implied. Further, such muscular action when it involves a change in body position is the description of the term *movement.* In fact, the *Dictionary of Education* defines motor activity as "movement accomplished by the contraction and relaxation of the muscles."[1] The human organism interacts with its environment through changes in position of the body and/or its segments through movement.

Movement is one of the most fundamental characteristics of life. Most of man's achievements are based upon his ability to move. Obviously, the very young child is not a highly intelligent being in the sense of abstract thinking, and he only gradually acquires the ability to deal with symbols and intellectualize his experience in the course of his development. Since the child is a creature of movement and feeling, any effort to educate him must take this dominance of movement into account.

Motor activity will be conceived throughout this text as things that children *do* actively in a pleasurable situation in order to learn. Generally speaking, these activities include (1) various

[1]Carter V. Good, *Dictionary of Education,* 2nd ed. New York, McGraw-Hill, Inc., 1959, p. 9.

3

forms of active games, (2) rhythmic activities and (3) stunt activities. In several of the subsequent chapters numerous examples of motor learning activites drawn from these three broad categories will be presented along with suggested applications for their use.

IMPORTANCE OF MOTOR ACTIVITY IN LEARNING

The idea of learning through motor activity is not necessarily new. In fact, the application of motor activity as a medium for learning was a basic principle of the Frobelian kindergarten early in the nineteenth century. It was based on the theory that children learn and acquire information, understanding and skills through motor activities in which they are naturally interested, such as building, constructing, modeling, painting and various forms of gross body movement. What perhaps *is* new is a unique and innovative application of this approach to learning, such as that suggested in the present text.

Another consideration is that much more attention is currently being paid to physical activity as an important aspect of the learning process. It cannot be stated unequivocally that there is an undisputed and widespread trend away from the traditional *sit still and listen* classroom environment. Nevertheless, more and more pronouncements by responsible individuals, in their descriptions of what constitutes a desirable learning environment for children, consistently reflect the importance of *physically-* oriented activities as invaluable kinds of learning experiences. Some representative examples of such statements follows.

In *The Relevance of Education,* Bruner elaborates upon his concept of the spiraling curriculum stating, "It has been true of various curriculum projects that their success depended upon the invention of appropriate embodiments of ideas in these three modes — in action, image, and symbol. The balance beam, the pendulum, the proper set of modular blocks, the well-designed game or role play . . . . these may be high technological achievements in education."[2]

---

[2]Jerome S. Bruner, *The Relevance of Education.* New York, W. W. Norton and Company, Inc., 1971, p. 122.

Murray presents evidence of several new kinds of intrinsic motives — sensory, curiosity, activity, manipulatory and cognitive which also relate to the *physical* aspect of the learner. He cites the *sensory deprivation* studies begun at McGill University which tend to refute those theories of motivation that hold that the organism basically seeks to reduce stimulation. While people may seek to avoid excessive environmental stimulation and inner tension, the students in the study found the state of nirvana intolerable. "They wanted stimulation so badly that they would ask to hear a recording of an old stock market report over and over again. Although they were asked to stay as long as possible, most subjects could take it for only two or three days. They preferred to work harder at less pay, in a stimulating environment."[3]

Behavior of the subjects during the sensory deprivation period was that of being unable to concentrate or sustain a train of thought after their intial attempts to think about personal and intellectual problems. They also had periods of confusion, irritability, stress and finally visual hallucinations. Such results might be correlated with behavior found in the sterile environment of some classrooms.

The curiosity motive was well demonstrated by the experiment with nursery school children.[4]

In this study the element of novelty and the intensity, color and complexity of the stimuli were found to be important variables that arouse interest of people. These elements might well be considered in the structuring of classroom activities.

In speaking of activity and manipulatory motives, Murray states, "a developing child is motivated to *do* things — to run, climb, throw, jump, hold, drop, open, and close."[5] Here the *physical* orientation of the young is also evident.

In Lee Bennett Hopkins' *Let Them Be Themselves*, which

---

[3]Edward J. Murray, Motivation and emotion. In Lazarus, Richard S. (Ed.): *Foundations of Psychology Series.* Englewood Cliffs, Prentice-Hall, Inc., 1964, p. 76.
[4]Edward J. Murray, Motivation and emotion. In Lazarus, Richard S. (Ed.): *Foundations of Psychology Series.* Englewood Cliffs, Prentice-Hall, Inc., 1964, p. 76.
[5]Edward J. Murray, Motivation and emotion. In Lazarus, Richard S. (Ed.): *Foundations of Psychology Series.* Englewood Cliffs, Prentice-Hall, Inc., 1964, p. 78.

serves as a useful storehouse of ideas for language arts enrichment activities, creative dramatics is presented as a means of facilitating language development and a readiness for reading.

"Thinking, daydreaming, imagining, playing, doing, and acting are all components of the art of being somewhere, something, or someone else. In the earliest years children's play is filled with acting. The block corner in the nursery and kindergarten is the place where young boys instantly become grown-up men — putting out fires, constructing bridges, . ."[6]

Hopkins goes on to state that "When children participate in dramatic play, they cooperate with one another, they begin to feel the need for exchanging ideas, they speak, they listen, their vocabularies improve, readiness for reading takes place, and pathways are opened to the direct teaching phases of written communication."[7]

Creative play enables children to bring the world of Cinderella, ogres, knights, and cops and robbers to have personal meaning through *physical* activity as they walk, talk, move, and react as these characters in the various situations they find themselves in.[8]

In outlining a variety of reading activities for an instructional program, Russell included "Creative activities growing out of reading to extend enjoyment or to reinforce the larger ideas of a selection or unit through dramatization, drawing a meaning, playing a game, or expressing ideas in rhythms."[9]

In an ESEA Title I project for oral language development of kindergarten and first grade children in the Syracuse City School System, action games along with experience stories and creative dramatics were activities used for providing drill in producing correct sounds. In the project the experimental group did significantly better than the control group when tested for oral communication skills. The increase in mean scores from the pretest and posttest results was about eighteen points for the experimental group in contrast to an approximately nine-point

---

[6]Lee Bennett Hopkins, *Let Them Be Themselves.* New York, Citation Press, 1969, p. 152.
[7]Lee Bennett Hopkins, *Let Them Be Themselves.* New York, Citation Press, 1969, p. 153.
[8]Lee Bennett Hopkins, *Let Them Be Themselves.* New York, Citation Press, 1969, p. 153.
[9]David H. Russell, *Children Learn to Read,* 2nd ed. New York, Ginn and Company, 1961, p. 145.

gain in the control group.

A very recent interesting phenomenon which relates to motor activity learning is concerned with what is called the *theory of bioplasmic forces*.[10] Briefly, this theory is based on the concept that all living matter is made up of an energy body and a physical body. Some educators hold to the belief that this theory of energy forces indicates that schools are wasting the energy needed for growth during the child's formative years by forcing premature intellectual learning of school subjects which could be more readily and easily mastered at a later age.[11] Moreover, certain studies in child and cognitive development suggest that academic learning before a child is maturationally ready will reduce his learning potential.[12] In this regard, the present author contends that the traditional procedures used to impose academic learning upon young children are not only incompatible with, but actually in violation of certain principles of child growth and development. (This point of view will be expounded extensively in the following chapter.)

THE THEORY OF CHILD LEARNING
THROUGH MOTOR ACTIVITY

The motor activity approach to learning is concerned with how children can develop skills and concepts in the various academic subject areas while actively engaged in any of the types of motor activities previously mentioned (an active game, stunt or rhythmic activity). It is based in part on the theory that children, being predominantly movement-oriented, will learn better when what might arbitrarily be called *academic learning* takes place through pleasurable physical activity; that is when the *motor* component operates at a maximal level in skill and concept

---

[10]For more details about this theory the reader is referred to the following source: Sheila Ostrander and Lynn Moore, *Psychic Discoveries Behind the Iron Curtain*. Englewood Cliffs, Prentice-Hall, Inc., 1971.

[11]Earl J. Ogletree, Intellectual growth in children and the theory of 'bioplasmic forces.' *Phi Delta Kappan*, February, 1974, p. 407.

[12]Raymond Moore, Robert Moon and Dennis Moore, The California report: Early schooling for all? *Phi Delta Kappan*, June, 1972, p. 617.

development in school subject areas essentially oriented to *verbal* learning. This is not to say that *motor* and *verbal* learning are two mutually exclusive kinds of learning, although it has been suggested that at the two extremes the dichotomy appears justifiable. It is recognized that in verbal learning which involves almost complete abstract symbolic manipulations there may be, among others, such motor components as tension, subvocal speech and physiological changes in metabolism which operate at a minimal level. It is also recognized that in motor activity where the learning is predominantly motor in nature, verbal learning is evident, although perhaps at a minimal level. For example, in teaching a motor activity there is a certain amount of verbalization in developing a kinesthetic concept of the particular activity that is being taught.

The procedure of learning through motor activity involves the selection of an activity such as an active game, stunt or rhythmic activity which is taught to the children and used as a learning activity for the development of a skill or concept in a specific subject area. An attempt is made to arrange an active learning situation so that a fundamental intellectual skill or concept is practiced or rehearsed in the course of participating in the motor activity.

Essentially, there are two general types of such activities. One type is useful for developing a specific concept where the learner *acts out* the concept and thus is able to visualize as well as to get the *feel* of the concept. Concepts become a part of the child's physical reality as the child participates in the activity where the concept is inherent. An example of such an activity follows.

The concept to be developed is the science concept *electricity travels along a pathway and needs a complete circuit over which to travel.* A motor activity in which this concept is inherent is *straddle ball roll.*

The children stand one behind the other in relay files with six to ten children in each file. All are in stride position with feet far enough apart so that a ball can be rolled between the legs of the players. The first person in each file holds a rubber playground ball. At a signal the person at the front of each file starts the activity by attempting to roll the ball between the legs of all the players on his team. The team which gets the ball to the last member of its file first in the manner described scores a point. The last player goes to the head of his file, and this procedure is continued with a point scored each time for the team that gets the ball back to the last player first. After every player has had an opportunity to roll the ball back the team which has scored the most points is declared the winner.

In applying this activity to develop the concept the first player at the head of each file becomes the electric switch which opens and shuts the circuit. The ball is the electric current. As the ball rolls between the children's legs it moves right through if all of the legs are properly lined up. When a leg is not in the proper stride, the path of the ball is impeded and the ball rolls out. The game has to be stopped until the ball is recovered and the correction made in the position of the leg. The circuit has to be repaired (the child's leg) before the flow of electricity (the roll of the ball) can be resumed.

The second type of activity helps to develop skills by using these skills in highly interesting and stimulating situations. Repetitive practice for the development of skills related to specific concepts can be utilized. An example of this type of activity follows.

This activity is an adaptation of the game *steal the bacon* and is used for practice on *initial consonants*. Children are put into two groups of seven each. The members of both teams are given the letters *b, c, d, h, m, n* and p, or any other initial consonants with which they have been having difficulty. The teams face each other about ten feet apart as in the following diagram.

b		p
c		n
d		m
h	beanbag (bacon)	h
m		d

n   c

p   b

The teacher calls out a word such as *ball*, and the two children having the letter *b* run out to grab the beanbag. If a player gets the beanbag back to his line, he scores two points for his team. If his opponent tags him before he gets back, the other team scores one point. The game ends when each letter has been called. The scores are totalled and the game is repeated with the children being identified with different letters.

TEACHING RESPONSIBILITY

It seems appropriate to take into account a very important aspect in the use of motor activity for learning. This is necessary because the motor activities used throughout this text derive from the kinds of experiences that are included in many physical education programs. This does *not* mean the use of motor activity for the development of academic skills and concepts takes place in the time allotted to physical education. On the contrary, this approach should be considered a learning activity in the same way other kinds of learning activities are used in a given subject area. This means that, for the most part, this procedure should be used during the time allotted to the particular subject area in question. Moreover, the classroom teacher would ordinarily do the teaching when this approach is used. The function of a physical education teacher could be to furnish the classroom teacher with suitable physical education activities to use in the development of concepts. This is to say that the classroom teacher is familiar with the skills and concepts to be developed, and similarly the physical education teacher should know those activities that could be adapted for use to develop the skills and concepts.

It has been the purpose of this introductory chapter to set forth an overview of the concept of learning through motor activity. The following chapter takes into account specific reasons why children tend to learn well through this medium.

CHAPTER TWO

FACTORS WHICH FACILITATE CHILD LEARNING THROUGH MOTOR ACTIVITY

DURING the early school years, and at ages six to eight particularly, it is likely that learning is limited frequently by a relatively short attention span rather than only by intellectual capabilities. Moreover, some children who do not appear to think or learn well in abstract terms can more readily grasp concepts when given an opportunity to use them in an applied manner. In view of the fact that the child is a creature of movement, and also that he is likely to deal better in concrete rather than abstract terms, it would seem to follow naturally that the motor activity learning medium is well suited for him.

The above statement should not be interpreted to mean that the author is suggesting that learning through movement-oriented experiences (motor learning) and passive learning experiences (verbal learning) are two different kinds of learning. The position is taken here that *learning is learning,* even though in the motor activity approach the motor component may be operating at a higher level than in most of the traditional types of learning activities.

The theory of learning accepted here is that learning takes place in terms of reorganization of the systems of perception into a functional and integrated whole because of the result of certain stimuli. This implies that problem solving is the way of desirable and worthwhile human learning and that learning takes place through problem solving. In a motor activity learning situation that is well planned, a great deal of consideration should be given to the inherent possibilities for learning in terms of problem solving. In this approach opportunities abound for near-ideal teaching-learning situations because of the many problems to be solved. Using active games as an example the following sample questions asked by children indicate that there is a great opportunity for reflective thinking, use of judgment and problem solving in this type of experience.

1. Why didn't I get to touch the ball more often?
2. How can we make it a better game?
3. Would two circles be better than one?
4. How can I learn to throw the ball better?

Another very important factor to consider with respect to the motor activity learning medium is that a considerable part of the learnings of young children are motor in character, with the child devoting a good proportion of his attention to skills of a locomotor nature. Furthermore, learnings of a motor nature tend to usurp a large amount of the young child's time and energy, and are often closely associated with other learnings. In addition, it is well known by experienced classroom teachers at the primary grade levels that the child's motor mechanism is active to the extent that it is almost an impossibility for him to remain for a very long period of time in a quiet state regardless of the passiveness of the learning situation.

To demand prolonged sedentary states of children is actually, in a sense, in defiance of a basic physiological principle. This is concerned directly with the child's basic metabolism. The term *metabolism* is concerned with physical and chemical changes in the body which involve producing and consuming energy. The rate at which these physical and chemical processes are carried on when the individual is in a state of rest represents his *basal metabolism*. Thus, the basal metabolic rate is indicative of the speed at which body fuel is changed to energy as well as how fast this energy is used.

Basal metabolic rate can be measured in terms of calories per meter of body surface, with a calorie representing a unit measure of heat energy in food. It has been found that, on the average, basal metabolism rises from birth to about two or three years of age, at which time it starts to decline until between the ages of twenty to twenty-four. Also, the rate is higher for boys than for girls. With the highest metabolic rate, and therefore the greatest amount of energy occurring during the early school years, deep consideration might well be given to learning activities through which this energy can be utilized. Moreover, it has been observed that there is an increased attention span of primary-age children during participation in active play. When a task such as a motor activity experience is meaningful to a child, he can spend longer periods engaged in it than is likely to be the case in some of the more traditional types of learning activities.

The comments made thus far have alluded to some of the *general* aspects of the value of the motor activity learning medium. The ensuing discussions will focus more specifically upon what might arbitrarily be called *inherent facilitative factors* in the motor activity learning medium which are highly compatible with child learning. These factors are *motivation, proprioception* and *reinforcement,* all of which are somewhat interdependent and interrelated.

MOTIVATION

In consideration of motivation as an inherent facilitative factor in learning through motor activity, the term should be thought of as it is described in the *Dictionary of Education* — that is "the practical art of applying incentives and arousing interest for the purpose of causing a pupil to perform in a desired way."[1]

One should also take into account *extrinsic* and *intrinsic* motivation. Extrinsic motivation is described as "the application of incentives that are external to a given activity to make work palatable and to facilitate performance," while intrinsic motivation is the "determination of behavior that is resident within an activity and that sustains it, as with autonomous acts and interests."[2]

Extrinsic motivation has been and continues to be used as a means of spurring individuals to achievement. This most often takes the form of various kinds of reward incentives. The main objection to this type of motivation is that it may tend to focus the learner's attention upon the reward rather than the learning task and the total learning situation.

[1]Carter V. Good, *Dictionary of Education,* 2nd edition. New York, McGraw-Hill, 1959, p. 354.
[2]Carter V. Good, *Dictionary of Education,* 2nd ed. New York, McGraw-Hill, 1959, p. 354.

In general, the child is motivated when he discovers what seems to him to be a suitable reason for engaging in a certain activity. The most valid reason of course is that he sees a purpose for the activity and derives enjoyment from it. The child must feel that what he is doing is important and purposeful. When this occurs and the child gets the impression that he is being successful in a group situation, the motivation is intrinsic: it comes about naturally as a result of the child's interest in the activity. It is the premise here that motor activity learning in the form of active games, stunts and rhythmic activities contain this *built in* ingredient so necessary to desirable and worthwhile learning.

The ensuing discussions of this section of the chapter will be concerned with three aspects of motivation that are considered to be inherent in the motor activity learning medium: (1) motivation in relation to *interest*, (2) motivation in relation to *knowledge of results*, and (3) motivation in relation to *competition*.

Motivation in Relation to Interest

It is important to have an understanding of the meaning of interest as well as an appreciation of how interests function as an adjunct to learning. As far as the meaning of the term is concerned, the following description given by Lee and Lee some time ago expresses in a relatively simple manner what is meant by the terms *interest* and *interests*. "Interest is a state of being, a way of reacting to a certain situation. Interests are those fields or areas to which a child reacts with interest consistently over an extended period of time."[3]

A good condition for learning is a situation in which a child agrees with and acts upon the learnings which he considers of most value to him. This means that the child accepts as most valuable those things that are of greatest interest to him. To the very large majority of children, pleasurable motor activity experiences are likely to be of the greatest personal value.

Under most circumstances a very high interest level is

[3]J. Murray Lee and Dorris May Lee, *The Child and His Development*, New York, Appleton-Century-Crofts, 1958, p. 382.

concomitant with pleasurable physical activities simply because of the expectation of pleasure children tend to associate with such activities. The structure of a learning activity is directly related to the length of time the learning act can be tolerated by the learner without loss of interest. Motor activity experiences by their very nature are more likely to be so structured than many of the traditional learning activities.

Motivation in Relation to Knowledge of Results

Knowledge of results is most commonly referred to as *feedback*. It was suggested by Brown many years ago that feedback is the process of providing the learner with information as to how accurate his reactions were.[4] Ammons has referred to feedback as knowledge of various kinds which the performer received about his performance.[5]

It has been reported by Bilodeau and Bilodeau that knowledge of results is the strongest, most important variable controlling performance and learning, and further, that studies have repeatedly shown that there is no improvement without it, progressive improvement with it, and deterioration after its withdrawal.[6] As a matter of fact, there appears to be a sufficient abundance of objective evidence that indicates that learning is usually more effective when one receives some immediate information on how he is progressing. It would appear rather obvious that such knowledge of results is an important adjunct to learning because one would have little idea of which of his responses was correct. Dolinsky makes the analogy that it would be like trying to learn a task while blindfolded.[7]

---

[4]J. S. Brown, A proposed program of research on psychological feedback (knowledge of results) in the performance of psychomotor tasks, Research Planning Conference on Perceptual and Motor Skills, AFHRRC Conf. Rept. 1949, U. S. Air Force, San Antonio, Texas, pp. 1-98.

[5]R. B. Ammons, Effects of knowledge of performance: A survey and tentative formulation, *J Gen Psych*, LIV: 279-99, 1956.

[6]Edward A. Bilodeau and Ina Bilodeau, Motor skill learning. *Annual Review of Psychology*. Palo Alto, California, 1961, pp. 243-270.

[7]Richard Dolinsky, *Human Learning*. Dubuque, Wm C. Brown Co., Publisher, 1966, p. 13.

The motor activity learning medium provides almost instantaneous knowledge of results because the child can actually *see* and *feel* himself throw a ball, or tag or be tagged in a game. He does not become the victim of a poorly constructed paper-and-pencil test, the results of which may have little or no meaning for him.

Motivation in Relation to Competition

Using active games as an example of motor activity to discuss the motivational factor of competition, one can arbitrarily describe games as *active interaction of children in cooperative and/or competitive situations*. It is possible to have both cooperation and competition functioning at the same time as in the case of team games. While one team is competing against the other, there is cooperation within each group. In this framework it could be said that a child is learning to cooperate while competing. It is also possible to have one group competing against another without cooperation within the group as in the case of games where all children run for a goal line independently and on their own.

The terms *cooperation* and *competition* are antonymous; therefore, the reconciliation of children's competitive needs and cooperative needs is not an easy matter. In a sense, one is confronted with an ambivalent condition, which if not carefully handled could place children in a state of conflict.

Modern society not only rewards one kind of behavior (cooperation), but also its direct opposite (competition). Perhaps more often than not our cultural demands sanction these rewards without provision of clear-cut standards with regard to specific conditions under which these forms of behavior might well be practiced. Hence, the child could be placed in somewhat of a quandary with regard to when to compete and when to cooperate.

In generalizing on the basis of the available evidence with regard to the subject of competition, it seems justifiable to formulate the following concepts.

1. Very young children in general are not very competitive but become more so as they grow older.

2. There is a wide variety in competition among children — that is some are violently competitive while others are mildly competitive, and still others are not competitive at all.

3. Boys tend to be more competitive than girls.

4. Competition should be adjusted so that there is not a preponderant number of winners over losers.

5. Competition and rivalry produce results in effort and speed of accomplishment.

In motor activity teaching-learning situations teachers might well be guided by the above concepts. As far as the competitive aspects of certain motor activities are concerned, they not only appear to be a good medium for learning because of the intrinsic motivation inherent in them, but this medium of learning can also provide for competitive needs of children in a pleasurable and enjoyable way.

PROPRIOCEPTION

Earlier in this chapter it was stated that the theory of learning accepted here is that learning takes place in terms of a reorganization of the systems of perception into a functional and integrated whole as a result of certain stimuli. These systems of perception, or sensory processes as they are sometimes referred to, are ordinarily considered to consist of the senses of sight, hearing, touch, smell and taste. Armington has suggested that "although this point of view is convenient for some purposes, it greatly over-simplifies the ways by which information can be fed into the human organism."[8] He indicates also that a number of sources of sensory input are overlooked, particularly the senses that enable the body to maintain its correct posture. As a matter of fact, the sixty or seventy pounds of muscle which include over six hundred in number that are attached to the skeleton of the averaged-sized man could well be his most important sense organ.

Various estimates indicate that the visual sense brings us more than three fourths of our knowledge. Therefore, it could be said

[8]John C. Armington, *Physiological Basis of Psychology*. Dubuque, Wm. C. Brown Co., Publisher, 1966, p. 16.

with little reservation that man is *eye-minded*. However, Steinhaus has reported that "a larger portion of the nervous system is devoted to receiving and integrating sensory input originating in the muscles and joint structures than is devoted to the eye and ear combined."[9] In view of this it could be contended that man is also *muscle sense* minded.

Generally speaking, *proprioception* is concerned with muscle sense. The proprioceptors are sensory nerve terminals that give information concerning movements and position of the body. A proprioceptive feedback mechanism is involved which in a sense regulates movement. In view of the fact that children are so movement-oriented, it appears a reasonable speculation that proprioceptive feedback from the receptors of muscles, skin and joints may contribute in a facilitative manner when the motor activity learning medium is used to develop academic skills and concepts. The combination of the psychological factor of motivation and the physiological factor of proprioception inherent in motor activity learning suggests the coining of the term *motorvation* to describe this phenomenon.

One writer has characterized the present author's concept in the following manner:

> Humphrey presents highly persuasive evidence for the effectiveness of his concepts. He suggests that sensory experiences arising from muscle action acts as a kind of coordinating process that aids in the integration of visual and auditory input, forming a holistic kind of perceptual experience as a child moves his body and limbs in the activities he has devised.[10]

REINFORCEMENT

In considering the compatibility of motor activity learning with reinforcement theory, the meaning of reinforcement needs to be taken into account. An acceptable general description of

---

[9]Arthur H Steinhaus, Your muscles see more than your eyes. *Journal of Health, Physical Education and Recreation*. September, 1966.

[10]Bryant J. Cratty, *Physical Expressions of Intelligence*. Englewood Cliffs, Prentice-Hall, 1972, p. 49.

reinforcement is that there is an increase in the efficiency of a response to a stimulus brought about by the concurrent action of another stimulus. The basis for contending that motor activity learning is consistent with general reinforcement theory is that this medium reinforces attention to the learning task and learning behavior. It keeps children involved in the learning activity, which is perhaps the major area of application for reinforcement procedures. Moreover, there is perhaps little in the way of human behavior that is not reinforced, or at least reinforcible, by feedback of some sort. The importance of proprioceptive feedback has already been discussed in this particular connection.

In summarizing this discussion, it would appear that motor activity learning generally establishes a more effective situation for learning reinforcement for the following reasons:

1. The greater motivation of the children in the motor activity learning situation involves accentuation of those behaviors directly pertinent to their learning activities, making these salient for the purpose of reinforcement.

2. The proprioceptive emphasis in motor activity learning involves a greater number of *responses* associated with and conditioned to learning stimuli.

3. The gratifying aspects of motor activity learning provide a generalized situation of *reinforcers*.

The first two chapters of this book have dealt generally with certain theoretical perspectives with regard to learning through motor activity. Any approach to teaching and learning should be based at least to some degree upon objective evidence produced by experimental research. This is the subject for discussion in the following chapter.

CHAPTER THREE.

RESEARCH IN CHILD LEARNING
THROUGH MOTOR ACTIVITY

THERE are a number of acceptable ways of studying how behavioral changes take place in children. After some amount of study and experimentation a certain sequence of techniques emerged as the most appropriate way to evaluate how well children might learn through motor activity. These techniques can generally be classified as follows:

1. Naturalistic Observation
2. Single-Group Experimental Procedure
3. Parallel-Group Experimental Procedure
4. Variations of Standard Experimental Procedures

NATURALISTIC OBSERVATION

One of the first problems to be reckoned with was whether this type of learning activity could be accomplished in the regular school situation and also whether teachers whose preparation and experience had been predominantly in traditional methods would subscribe to this particular approach. To obtain this information, a procedure that could best be described as *naturalistic observation* was used. This involved the teaching of a skill or concept in a particular subject area to a group of children and using a motor activity in which the skill or concept was inherent. The teacher would then evaluate how well the skill or concept was learned through the motor activity learning medium. The teacher's criteria for evaluation were his or her past experiences with other groups of children and other learning media. Two representative *cases* of the process of naturalistic observation follow. Each contains a statement of the concept to be developed, the activity and a specific application of it, and an evaluation by the teacher.

Case 1

Concept: Things which are balanced have equal weights on either side of their central point.

Activity: RUSH AND TUG. This is a combative activity in which the class is divided into two groups with each group standing behind one of two parallel lines which are about forty feet apart. In the middle of these two parallel lines a rope is laid perpendicular to them. A cloth is tied in the middle of the rope to designate the halves of the rope. On a signal, members of both groups rush to their respective ends of the rope, pick it up and tug toward the group's end line. The group pulling the midpoint of the rope past its own endline in a specified amount of time is declared the winner. If at the end of the designated time the midpoint of the rope has not been pulled beyond one group's endline, the group with the midpoint of the rope nearer to its endline is declared the winner.

Application: In performing this combative activity it was decided to have the groups experiment with all kinds of combinations of teams such as boys versus boys, girls versus girls, boys versus girls, big ones against little ones, and mixed sizes and weights against the same.

Evaluation: This was a very stimulating experience for the group since it presented to them a genuine problem-solving situation in trying to get the exact combination of children for an equal balance of the two teams. When there was enough experimenting, two teams of equal proportions were assembled. It was found that it was most difficult for either to make any headway. They also discovered that an equal balance depended not only on the weight of their classmates, but to some extent upon their strength as well. Other classes where the motor activity learning medium had not been used had shown much less interest in this concept. It was speculated that this was perhaps due to the fact that the procedure presented problem-solving situations that were of immediate interest and concern to the children in a concrete manner.

Case 2

Concept: We divide to find how many groups there are in a larger group.

Activity: GET TOGETHER. Players take places around the activity area in a scattered formation. The leader calls any number by which the total number of players is not exactly divisible. All players try to form groups of the number called. Each group joins hands in a circle. The one or ones left out have points scored against them. Low score wins the game.

Application: If there are twenty-three players in the group and the teacher calls out the number 7, the players try to run to form groups of seven. There would be a remainder of 2. Depending upon the age and ability level of the children, various numbers can be called.

Evaluation: In one particular instance a teacher-evaluation indicated that this activity was useful for reinforcing the idea of groups or sets and that groups are of like things (in this case children). It gave the children the idea that there may be a *remainder* when dividing into groups.

Naturally, this procedure is grossly lacking in objectivity because there is only a subjective evaluation of the teacher to support the hypothesis. However, in the early stages of the work this technique served the purpose well because at that time the main concern was having teachers experiment with the idea, and to ascertain their reaction to it. In a vast majority of cases the reactions of teachers were very positive.

SINGLE GROUPS

The next factor that needed to be taken into consideration was whether or not children could *actually* learn through the motor activity learning medium. Although for centuries empirical evidence had placed the hypothesis in a very positive position, there was still the need for some objective evidence to support the hypothesis. In order to determine if learning could actually take place through motor activity, the *single group technique* was employed. This technique involved the criterion measure of objective pretesting of a group of children on certain skills or concepts in a given subject area. Motor activities in which the skills or concepts were involved were taught to the children over a specified period of time and used as learning activities to develop the skills or concepts. After the specified period of time the children were retested and served as their own controls for comparing results of the posttest with the results of the pretest.

All of the studies involving this technique in which the subjects were their own controls have shown significant differences between pretest and postest scores at a very high level of probability. Therefore, it appeared reasonable to generalize that learning actually could take place through the motor activity learning medium.

PARALLEL GROUPS

With the preceding information at hand, the next and obviously the most important step in the sequence of research techniques was to attempt to determine how the motor activity learning medium compared with other more traditional media. For this purpose the *parallel group technique* was used. This involved pretesting children on a number of skills or concepts in a given subject area and equating them into groups. One group was designated as the motor activity group (experimental group), and an attempt made to develop the skills or concepts through the motor activity learning medium. The other group was designated as the traditional group (control group), and an attempt made to develop the skills or concepts through one or more traditional media. Both groups were taught by the same classroom teacher over a specified period of time. At the end of the experiment both groups were retested and comparisons were made of the posttest scores of both groups.

VARIATIONS OF STANDARD
EXPERIMENTAL PROCEDURES

Along with the above, a number of variations of standard techniques have been employed. In studying the effectiveness of the motor activity learning medium for boys compared to girls, a procedure was used that involved parallel groups of boys and girls within the total single group.

In those cases where an attempt has been made to hold a certain specific variable constant, three groups have been used. In this situation one group becomes an observing or nonparticipating group.

Another variation has been to equate children into two groups with each group taught by a different teacher. This can be done for the purpose of comparing a physical education teacher who would not likely be skilled in teaching concepts in another curriculum area with a superior classroom teacher who would likely be highly skilled in this direction.

In most of the studies the experiment is carried on over a period of ten days. (In some cases where conditions permit, this time period has been longer.) There are ordinarily eight and sometimes as many as ten skills or concepts involved. A ten-day period allows for two days of testing and eight days of teaching. Reliability for the objective tests has ordinarily been obtained by using a test-retest with similar groups of children. All of the experiments have been done in the actual school situation. Obviously, it would be better to carry them out over extended periods of time, but in most cases it has been impractical to do so because it usually involves some interruption in the regular school program. In addition, it should be mentioned that these studies are much more exploratory than they are definitive; this is ordinarily the case when conducting almost any kind of research where young children are involved.

SOME REPRESENTATIVE RESEARCH FINDINGS

Over a period of about twenty years a relatively large number of studies have been carried out utilizing the various techniques reported previously. Following are some representative examples of these studies in the areas of reading, mathematics and science. (An extensive bibliography of research conducted or directed by the author appears as an Appendix.)

Reading

The first experiment reported here involved a detailed study of the reactions of six to eight-year-old children when independent reading material is oriented to active game participation.[1] This experiment was initiated on the premise of relating reading content for six to eight-year-old children to their natural urge to play.

Ten games were written with a story setting. The original manuscripts were very carefully prepared. Care was given to the reading values and the literary merits of each story. Attention was focused upon (1) particular reading skills, (2) concept development, (3) vocabulary load in terms of the number, repetition and difficulty of words, and (4) length, phrasing and number of sentences per story.

After the manuscripts were prepared, the *New Readability Formula for Grades I-III* by George D. Spache was applied to judge the reading difficulty of the material. Application of this formula revealed the following results.

READING DIFFICULTY OF THE GAME STORIES
BASED ON THE SPACHE FORMULA

Factors Inherent in the Stories	*Range*	*Median*	*Mean*
Number of words per story	56-143	103.5	96.8
Number of sentences per story	8-24	15.5	15.6
Number of words per sentence	4.9-7.1	6.5	6.2
Grade level of readability	1.6-2.2	1.85	1.85

A total of 968 words was used in the stories. Eleven of these words, or about 1 percent, were *not* included in the *Clarence H. Stone's Revision of the Dale List of 769 Easy Words,* the word list used in the Spache Formula.

After the Spache Readability Formula was applied, thirty teachers in rural, suburban and city school systems working with fifty-four reading groups of children used and evaluated the stories in actual classroom situations. The reading groups varied

---

[1]James H. Humphrey and Virginia D. Moore, Improving reading through physical education. *Education* (The Reading Issue), May, 1960, p. 559.

in (1) number, from 3 to 33; (2) chronological age, from five years, nine months to nine years, eight months; (3) intelligence quotient, from 52 to 136; and (4) grade placement, from first grade to third grade. The children represented to a reasonable extent a cross section of an average population with respect to ethnic background, socioeconomic level and the like. In all, 503 children read from one to three stories for a total of 1,007 different readings.

On report sheets especially designed for the purpose the teachers were asked to record observable evidence of certain comprehension skills being practiced by the reading groups. The teachers were requested to make their evaluations on a comparative basis with other materials that had been read by the children. The results of these observations follows.

COMPREHENSION SKILLS PRACTICED BY
CHILDREN AS OBSERVED BY TEACHERS

Comprehension Skill	*Number of Groups Observed*	*Number and Percent of Groups Practicing Skills*
Following directions	54	49-91%
Noting and using sequence of ideas	54	41-76%
Selecting main idea	54	41-76%
Getting facts	54	36-67%
Organizing ideas	54	25-46%
Building meaningful vocabulary	54	22-41%
Gaining independence in word mastery	54	19-35%

The observations of the teachers indicated that the game stories gave the children opportunities to practice and maintain skills necessary for intelligent reading. While enriching and extending their experiences, the children improved their general ability to read independently and *on their own.*

In another dimension of the study teachers were asked to rate the degree of *interest* of the children in the reading on an arbitrary five-point scale as follows: extreme interest, considerable interest, moderate interest, some interest, or little or no interest. Again the teachers established their own criteria in rating for degree of interest.

The fact that there was sustained interest in the game stories is shown by the following. (The 25 cases in the last two categories involved children with intelligence quotients far below normal.)

DEGREE OF INTEREST IN THE READING AS RATED BY TEACHERS

Degree of Interest	Number of Cases	Number and Percent of Cases
Extreme interest	1,007	469-46%
Considerable interest	1,007	242-24%
Moderate interest	1,007	271-27%
Some interest	1,007	22-2.7%
Little or no interest	1,007	3- .3%

This dimension of the study tended to show that reading was an active rather than a passive process. Apparently the children had a real and genuine purpose for reading, to satisfy the natural urge to play they were *interested* and read to learn a new game.

It would certainly be hazardous to make sweeping generalizations on the basis of the results of this study. This comment is made because of the great interest teachers expressed as a result of their observations. In fact, some seemed to view the procedure as a possible panacea for most of the reading problems that occur in the school situation. However, caution should be observed in drawing conclusions. On the basis of the findings of this study and within the limitations involved in conducting such an experiment, the following generalizations appear warranted.

1. When a child is self-motivated and interested, he reads. In this case the reading was done without the usual motivating devices such as picture clues and illustrations. Certainly illustrations with reading materials at this age level are important.

2. These game stories were found to be extremely successful in stimulating interest in reading and, at the same time, improving the child's ability to read.

3. Because the material for these game stories was scientifically selected, prepared and tested, it is unique in the field of children's independent reading material. The outcomes were most satisfactory in terms of children's interest in reading content of this nature as well as motivation to read.

In the next study reported here, 20 third grade children were equated into two groups on the basis of pretest scores on ten language understandings.[2] One group was taught through motor activities in the form of active games. The other group was taught through traditional language workbooks. Both groups had the same teacher. Comparisons were made of the pretest and posttest scores of the language workbook group and also the active game group. The statistical analysis showed that both groups learned, but that the active game groups learned at a higher level of significance. When the posttest scores of both groups were analyzed, it was indicated that the active game group learned significantly more than the language workbook group.

In recognition of the limitations imposed by a study of this nature, it was generalized that if one accepts the significant differences in the test scores as evidence of learning, these third-grade children could develop language comprehension through both active games and the traditional language workbook medium, although the active game medium produced greater changes.

The final reading study reported here was designed to evaluate the effectiveness of active games as a means of reinforcing reading skills with fourth grade children.[3] The purpose of this study was to determine how well certain reading skills could be reinforced by motor activity in the form of active games as compared with some of the traditional ways of reinforcing these skills.

Seventy-three fourth grade children were pretested on eight reading skills. Thirty of these children were divided into two groups. One group of fifteen was designated as the active game

[2] James H. Humphrey, Comparison of the use of active games and language workbook exercises as learning media in the development of language understanding with third grade children. *Perceptual and Motor Skills, 21*:23, 1965.

[3] James H. Humphrey, The use of the active game learning medium in the reinforcement of reading skills with fourth-grade children. *The Journal of Special Education, 1*:369, 1967.

group and the other group of fifteen as the traditional group. Each reading skill was introduced and presented verbally to the two groups together. The groups were then separated, and with one group the reading skills were reinforced through various forms of active games. With the other group the reading skills were reinforced by such traditional media as a language workbook, a dictionary and prepared ditto sheets. Both groups were taught by the same teacher. The types of reading skills used in the study were structural analysis, phonics, word recognition and vocabulary development.

After the reading skills were presented in the manner described, both groups were retested. The experiment covered ten school days, allowing one day for pretesting, eight days for the experiment, and a final day for posttesting. A comparison of the posttest mean scores showed that the active game group learned significantly more than the traditional group. Therefore, it was concluded that the kinds of reading skills used in this study could be reinforced to better advantage by active games than by some more traditional approaches.

Mathematics

The first study in the area of mathematics reported here is an example of a single group experimental procedure with parallel groups of boys and girls within the single group.[4] The purpose of this study was to determine how well a group of first grade children might develop number concepts through motor activity in the form of active games, and at the same time to ascertain whether the approach was more favorable for boys or for girls.

Thirty-five first grade children were pretested on eight number concepts which were to be included as a part of their regular class work during the ensuing two weeks. Ten boys and ten girls who had the same pretest scores were selected for the experiment. Eight active games in which the number concepts were involved and which were appropriate for use at first grade level were selected.

The active games were taught to the twenty children and used

[4]James H. Humphrey, An exploratory study of active games in learning of number concepts by first grade boys and girls, *Perceptual and Motor Skills*, 23, 1966.

as learning media for the development of the number concepts. They were retested after the active game medium was used. The scores of the first test for all of the twenty children ranged from 30 to 73, and the scores on the second test from 59 to 78. The mean score of the first test was 51.7 and the mean score of the second test was 68. In computing the results for the ten boys and the ten girls separately, the mean scores for the second test for the boys was 70.5 and for the girls, 65.5. The statistical analysis showed that as a total single group there was a highly significant difference from pretest to posttest mean scores. In comparing boys with girls, the results indicated greater changes in learning were produced with the boys.

For a clearer picture of the direction of differences between the boys and girls, the percentages of differences in gain on a paired per pupil basis follow.

Subject Pair	Differences in % of Gain	Sex
1	0	
2	11	Boy
3	0	
4	8	Girl
5	41	Boy
6	40	Boy
7	31	Boy
8	34	Boy
9	64	Boy
10	28	Girl

Six of the boys had a greater percentage difference in gain than the girls, while two of the girls had a greater percentage difference in gain. In two cases there was no difference.

In the next study reported here, a large number of pupils were involved in a comparison of motor activity learning by active games with two other procedures in developing concepts related to the telling of time.[5]

Forty-two classes of third grade pupils, for a total of 1,147 children from eighteen school districts were used as subjects in this study. The original parent population from which the forty-two classes were randomly selected consisted of 319 third grade classes from 166 elementary schools.

The forty-two classes were divided into three groups of fourteen each. One group was taught through the developmental-meaningful method. A second group was taught through the drill method, and with the third group the active game approach was used. All classes were taught by their own classroom teacher.

Three sets of lesson plans, one for each group, were devised. Instructions to the teachers were included in each set of lesson plans. Lesson plans for the developmental-meaningful group closely followed the objectives, suggested activities and problems used in the several textbooks most prevalent in the area. Lesson plans for the drill group and active game group paralleled the materials covered in the developmental-meaningful group. In the lesson plans for the drill group, the suggestions took the form of having the pupils work prepared examples in individual drill booklets. In the lesson plans for the active game group, the suggestions took the form of pleasurable active games. A twelve-foot clock was painted on the playground of each school, using the active game procedure, and materials needed for the implementation of the program were made available. Included in this equipment were four playground balls, two sets of flash cards, and one set of numbered blocks.

There were ten teaching days in the experiment. All teachers were to teach each lesson in twenty-minute periods. A lesson began immediately after the teacher had read the stated objectives for the current lesson. All teachers taught the time-telling lesson at the same time each day. Teachers who used the active game approach considered time spent on lesson plans for this

[5]Thomas Crist, A comparison of the use of the active game learning medium with developmental-meaningful and drill procedures in developing concepts for telling time at third-grade level. Doctoral dissertation, University of Maryland, College Park, Maryland, 1968.

experiment as part of their arithmetic class rather than part of their physical education time.

Two parallel forms (Forms A and B) of a performance test in time-telling concepts were constructed and used as criterion measures for the study. Each form of the criterion measure contained seventy-four items divided into two main parts. Part I of each form consisted of sixty items purported to measure primarily a basic understanding of time-telling and the comprehension of the passing time. Part II of each form consisted of fourteen verbal problems. Form A was administered as a pretest and form B as a posttest.

In comparing the pretest and posttest of each individual group as its own control, it was indicated that all groups learned significantly from pretest to posttest. However, the highest level of probability was shown in the active game group; the second highest, in the developmental-meaningful group; and the lowest, in the drill group. When a comparison was made of the posttest scores of all three groups, there was no significant difference between any of the three groups. In view of the fact that none of the teachers taking part in the experiment had ever taught an academic concept through the use of motor activity, it seemed reasonable to consider that any conclusions drawn must necessarily take this factor into account. It was also necessary to assume that all of the teachers had some, if not a considerable amount of preparation and experience in the use of the developmental-meaningful and drill-teaching procedures. Therefore, it would appear justifiable to speculate what results would have been obtained if a similar experiment could be carried out using teachers with a motor activity-oriented teacher-preparation background to teach time-telling on the playground instead of teachers with only a general elementary education background. Further, because paper-and-pencil tests were used, the whole experimental testing procedure could be said to be slanted toward the two traditional classroom procedures. Again, one could speculate as to the results if the testing (posttesting) had been administered under one of the following circumstances: (1) testing the pupils in all three procedures in an active game locale, (2) testing the pupils taught by the active game procedures with a paper-and-pencil test and testing pupils taught by the developmental-meaningful and drill procedures in an active game situation, and (3) testing pupils taught by the active game procedure in an active game locale and testing pupils taught by the other two procedures with a paper-and-pencil test.

The final study in mathematics reported here attempted to determine whether or not motor learning activities could be used as a practical and effective enrichment aid in the teaching of selected first grade mathematical concepts.[6]

Two units of the Book I program of a standard mathematics series were reviewed, and ten concepts selected. From these concepts, an objective test containing five items per concept was developed. Each item was rated for difficulty, and questions which received a score below .30 and above .75 on the difficulty rating were reworded.

The test was administered to the subject class and using the results of this pretest, the subject class was divided into two equal groups. Motor activity learning experiences were then selected to enrich each of the mathematical concepts.

The *entire* class received traditional classroom teaching procedures in learning the mathematical concepts involved. After each lesson, the enrichment group (experimental group) was given enrichment by the physical education teacher through the use of a variety of physical education activities. The control group participated in free play supervised by the classroom teacher during this time.

After four weeks of the above procedure, a posttest was administered to both groups. After an additional four weeks without enrichment, an extended interval test was administered to both groups.

In comparing the pretest scores, no significant differences were found between the groups as a whole and for each sex separately. Significant differences were found at a very high level of probability between the scores of the posttest for the groups as a

---

[6]Frank, Krug, The use of physical education activities in the enrichment of learning of selected first-grade mathematical concepts. Master's thesis, University of Maryland, College Park, Maryland, 1973.

whole and for each sex separately, with the enrichment group learning more than the control group. Comparing the extended interval tests, no significant differences were found between groups for girls and boys separately; however, when considered as an entire group, significance was found at a high level of probability favoring the enrichment group.

Further interpretations of the data indicated that the results of the pretest showed that both control and enrichment groups started out statistically equal. This was observed for all groups (girls only, boys only, and boys and girls combined.) The results of the posttest showed that all control and enrichment groups learned the mathematical concepts at a very high level of probability. The results of the posttest further showed that all enrichment groups learned significantly more than the control groups. The results of the extended interval tests showed that all groups retained what they had learned. The enrichment group more effectively retained their learning over the control group when examined as boys and girls combined.

In addition to the statistical analysis, the following subjective evaluation was made by the cooperating classroom teacher:

> The children had difficulty understanding why only half of them went with their physical education teacher after mathematics. By this, I mean the enrichment group felt privileged while the control group felt left out. However, they came to accept this after a few days. Those who were in the enrichment group looked forward to going with the physical education teacher. They enjoyed the games immensely. Now that the experiment is completed, the children in the enrichment group have shown me many of the games they played with the physical education teacher and how they related to the concepts being taught in class. We are now using some of the games as reinforcement for other concepts. I have found this extremely beneficial. In my estimation, the experiment was well-planned, well-conducted, and of value to the children.

Generalizations drawn from this study were that the use of motor learning activities was effective in enriching the mathematical concepts involved and should be considered as an enrichment aid when teaching first grade mathematical concepts.

Further, the classroom teacher recommended that physical education teachers might well be considered as important consultants in the planning of certain types of learning experiences relevant to first grade mathematical concepts. In other words, the physical education teacher could be considered as a valuable co-worker with the classroom teacher in the development of mathematical concepts.

Science

The first study in the area of science reported here is one in which the parallel group procedure was used. The purpose of this study was to compare the use of the motor activity learning medium with traditional teaching procedures in the development of selected fifth grade science concepts.[7] In this study the science concepts were equated rather than the children. The reason for this was that an experiment that involved the equating of children would have caused too much confusion in the particular school situation where the experiment was carried out.

Seventy-two fifth grade science concepts were collected from a variety of sources which included courses of study, representative fifth grade science textbooks, and a number of science concepts charts. The concepts were organized into a scale and rated by a jury of ten educators on the basis of how *difficult* they were to develop with an average fifth grade class. The jury consisted of five educators whose functions were of an administrative or supervisory nature and five teachers of elementary school science judged superior by their supervisors. From the twenty concepts rated the most difficult to develop with an average fifth grade class, nine were selected that possibly could have been developed through a motor learning activity as well as through traditional procedures. Questions testing for knowledge of these concepts were developed and checked as to validity by means of a jury appraisal technique. Nine motor learning activities were selected

---

[7]Charles F. Ison, An experimental study of a comparison of the use of physical education activities as a learning medium with traditional procedures in the development of selected fifth-grade science concepts. Master's thesis, University of Maryland, College Park, Maryland, 1961.

to use as learning activities for developing nine of the eighteen science concepts. Traditional procedures were used to teach the remaining nine concepts. The eighteen science concepts were taught in this manner by two fifth grade teachers in separate schools. One science period was used to teach each concept, and the two methods by which the concepts were developed were alternated. No significant difference was found between the posttest scores of the concepts that were taught through the different methods. Significant differences were found at a high level of probability in both classes between pretest and posttest scores of the concepts taught through the motor activity learning medium. This condition existed in only one of the classes taught through traditional procedures. However, it could only be concluded that both procedures provided valid learning experiences for these particular groups. A factor strongly favoring the motor activity learning medium was that the classroom teachers' preparation and experience had been with the traditional procedures rather than with the motor activity learning medium.

The next study involved the reinforcement or enrichment of science concepts through motor activity.[8] Twenty-three first grade children were pretested on a science unit on simple machines. The children were equated into two groups on the basis of the pretest. The classroom teacher taught eight science lessons to the entire class of twenty-three children to illustrate eight first grade science concepts involving simple machines. The teacher used regular traditional teaching procedures with the class.

Immediately after each science lesson the physical education teacher took eleven of the children (experimental group) on the basis of the pretest scores and attempted to reinforce the concepts through various kinds of physical education activities. The other twelve children (control group) took part in such activities as art work or story-telling with the classroom teacher. These activities of the control group were not related to the science concepts.

---

[8]Iris J. Prager, The use of physical education activities in the reinforcement of selected first-grade science concepts. Master's thesis, University of Maryland, College Park, Maryland, 1968.

After the procedure was followed for a two-week period, all of the children were retested. The results of this posttest showed that the group whose learning was reinforced by the physical education teacher through motor activities was significantly greater than the group not reinforced by such procedures. In comparing each group separately as its own control, it was indicated that the group reinforced by the motor activity medium gained significantly at a very high level of probability while the other group did not improve significantly. The results also showed that the reinforcement procedure was more favorable for boys than for girls at this age level.

On the basis of the results of this study, the following generalizations appeared warranted:

1. The activities taught by the physical education teacher should be considered as a reinforcement aid in teaching first grade science concepts.

2. This procedure should be given consideration in developing science concepts with first grade boys because the results were so favorable to learning for boys.

3. The physical education teacher might well be considered an important consultant in the planning of certain types of learning experiences in the science curriculum.

In the final study on science reported here two groups of slower learning fifth grade children were equated on the basis of pretest scores on science concepts.[9] One group was designated as the motor activity group and the other as the traditional group. The IQ range of the motor activity group was 74 to 89, with a mean of 85. The traditional group's IQ range was from 72 to 90, with a mean of 83. The children were tested three times. After the first test had been administered to a large group, two groups of ten each were selected. Both groups were taught the same science concepts by the same classroom teacher, one through traditional procedures and the other through the motor activity learning medium. The teaching was over a two-week period at which time

[9]James H. Humphrey, The use of motor activity learning in the development of science concepts with slow learning fifth-grade children. *Journal of Research in Science Teaching, 9*: No. 3, 1972.

the children were retested. Following this second test there was no formal instruction on the science concepts that were taught during this two-week period. They were tested a third time at an interval of three months after the second test. The following arrays of scores show the results of all three tests for all children.

	Traditional Group				Motor Activity Group		
Pupil	*Test 1*	*Test 2*	*Test 3*	*Pupil*	*Test 1*	*Test 2*	*Test 3*
A	43	23	40	A	43	73	73
B	23	43	43	B	23	60	67
C	37	33	37	C	37	63	73
D	50	63	60	D	50	73	90
E	53	63	50	E	53	73	83
F	47	57	60	F	47	60	70
G	47	47	53	G	47	77	63
H	33	53	40	H	33	60	67
I	50	77	63	I	50	90	87
J	33	43	57	J	33	70	60
Total	416	502	503	*Total*	416	699	733
Mean	41.6	50.2	50.3	*Mean*	41.6	69.9	73.3

The difference in mean scores was used as the criterion for learning. When analyzed statistically, it was found that the motor activity group learned significantly more than the traditional group. Also, the motor activity group showed a higher level of retention for the three-month period. Although the traditional group retained what was learned, the gain in learning was minimal to begin with.

In addition to the quantitative data reported above, there was observable evidence of many more opportunities for reasoning and problem-solving in the experiences of the motor activity group than for the group taught by the traditional procedures.

SOME GENERALIZATIONS OF THE RESEARCH FINDINGS

It should be mentioned again that the research in this general area is much more exploratory than definitive. However, it is interesting to note that no study has shown a significant difference in traditional procedures over the motor activity learning procedure.

In view of the fact that there are now some objective data to at least partially support a long-held hypothetical postulation, perhaps some generalized assumptions along with some reasonable speculations can be set forth with some degree of confidence. Obviously, the available data are not extensive enough to carve out a clear-cut profile with regard to learning through motor activity. However, they are suggestive enough to give rise to some interesting generalizations which may be briefly summarized as follows:

1. In general, children tend to learn certain academic concepts better through the motor activity learning medium than through many of the traditional media.

2. This approach, while favorable for both boys and girls, appears to be more favorable for boys.

3. The approach appears to be more favorable for children with average and below average intelligence.

4. For children with high levels of intelligence, it may be possible to introduce more advanced concepts at an earlier age through the motor activity learning medium.

It will remain the responsibility of further research to provide more conclusive evidence to support these generalizations and speculations. There is hope, however, based on actual experience with this approach in the activities described throughout this text, and particularly in Chapters Five through Nine, to encourage those responsible for facilitating child learning of academic concepts to use this approach and to join in collecting evidence to verify the contribution of motor activity learning to the education curriculum.

CHAPTER FOUR

IMPORTANCE OF MOTOR ACTIVITY
LEARNING FOR SLOW LEARNERS

IT will perhaps be recalled that one of the important research findings reported in the previous chapter was concerned with the positive effect of motor activity learning on slow-learning children. Perhaps the primary reason for this is that slow learners do not necessarily tend to deal as well with the more abstract kinds of learning situations inherent in many of the traditional school procedures. On the contrary, the motor activity learning medium involves a much more meaningful kind of experience for the child. The learning environment is such that the child actually has a direct, purposeful and pleasurable experience when participating in a motor activity.

In recent times many of the various curriculum areas have demonstrated an interest in body movement as an important adjunct to learning for the low achiever. This idea has been particularly pronounced in the area of elementary school science. Tangible evidence of this concern is reflected in the fact that the National Science Teachers Association at its national convention in 1973 inaugurated a session specifically oriented to the needs of children who have difficulty in learning. This session was called "Science for the Mentally Handicapped." The success of this session prompted its continuance at the national convention of 1974. This session was called "Science in Special Education." This session involved presentations and discussions on instructional problems with emphasis on activities that are adaptable to special education situations. Evidence of the interest in the motor activity approach was indicated by an invitation of the present author to address both of these sessions.[1, 2]

[1]James H. Humphrey, The use of motor activity in the development of science concepts with mentally handicapped children. Proceedings, Twenty First National Convention of the National Science Teachers Association, Washington, D. C., 1973.

The basic principle of *teaching to the individual differences of the learner* has led to the development of many components within the educational system. Programs and services are becoming available in school systems that reflect the needs of those with widely varying abilities and interests. Programs and services are being directed to serving citizens of all ages, beginning with the nursery-kindergarten, and extending to adult education classes.

Within this broad concept of educational opportunities for our nation's population, there has developed a national concern in recent years for the problems of children with learning impairment. Direct grants for research and service for these children have enabled government agencies and private foundations to work cooperatively to help the schools do a better job, both in identifying these children and providing more appropriate learning environments for them. The neurologist, the physician, the psychologist and the researcher in education are contributing new insights into working with these children.

Some of the research in ways children with mental deficits and impairment learn provides the teacher with useful guidelines. Research has been directed not only to the etiology, the nature and the degree of learning impairment, but also to the educational environment within which learning takes place for children with such impairment. It is the premise of the author that the approach to learning through active physical involvement of the learner is one that needs more recognition and greater emphasis in the learning environment of those children who are identified as *slow learners.*

IDENTIFYING THE SLOW LEARNER

While there has been agreement that the needs of children with learning impairment must be reflected in appropriate teaching techniques, there is an increasing awareness of the problems of identification. Too many children in our classrooms have been

---

[2]James H. Humphrey, Developing science concepts with slow learning children through active games. Proceedings, Twenty Second National Convention of the National Science Teachers Association, Washington, D. C., 1974.

mistaken for slow learners because of their difficulties in mastering such academic skills as reading and arithmetic. It is essential, therefore, that there can be a clear understanding of basic differences among children with the *slow learner syndrome*, but whose learning problems may be caused by factors other than subnormal intellectual functioning. With this general frame of reference in mind, the subsequent discussions will focus upon slow learners classified as (1) the child with mental retardation, (2) the child with depressed potential and (3) the child with a learning disability.

The Child With Mental Retardation

In the literature the broad generic term *mentally retarded* encompasses all degrees of mental deficit. The designation of the term *slow learner* has been given to those children who have a mild degree (along a continuum) of subnormal intellectual functioning as measured by intelligence tests. The intelligence quotients of these children fall within the range of 70 or 75 to 90. This child in the classroom is making average or below average progress in the academic skills, depending where he falls along the continuum of mental retardation. He will probably demonstrate slowness in learning such academic skills as reading and possibly arithmetic. He will very likely have difficulty in the area of the more complex mental processes of defining, analyzing and comparing. He tends to be a poor reasoner. However, he need not necessarily be equally slow in all aspects of behavior. He may be above average in social adaptability or artistic endeavors.

In respect to physical characteristics, personality and adjustment, slow-learning children are as variable and heterogeneous as children in the average and above-average range of intellectual potential. Attributes often identified with slow learners are laziness, inattention and short attention. However, these characteristics are likely to be eliminated when the educational environment is geared to the needs of children and when there is appropriateness, meaningfulness and purposefulness to the learning activity.

There is some variance in the literature as to whether these children should be identified as mentally retarded. There is general agreement that the slow learner represents a mild degree of subnormal intellectual functioning, whether or not he is labeled mentally retarded. Kirk has described the characteristic educational life patterns of those within the broad educational categories of subnormal intelligence, namely (a) the slow learner, (b) the educable mentally retarded, (c) the trainable mentally retarded, and (d) the totally dependent mentally retarded. With reference to the slow learner he states.

> The slow-learning child is not considered mentally retarded because he is capable of achieving a moderate degree of academic success even though at a slower rate than the average child. He is educated in the regular class program without special provisions except an adaptation of the regular class program to fit his slower learning ability. At the adult level he is usually self-supporting, independent and socially adjusted.[3]

In recent years the dimension of social adaptiveness has gained as an influencing criterion for identification of the mentally retarded. Dywab discusses the criterion of *social acceptance.* He speaks of the growing reluctance to identify persons as mentally retarded on the basis of intellectual subnormality alone.

Thus, a man who scores 65 on an intelligence test and who at the same time shows himself well able to adapt to the social demands of his particular environment at home, at work and in the community should not be considered retarded. Indeed, it is now known that he is not generally so considered.[4]

It is apparent, therefore, that the slow learner with whom the teacher may be working in the classroom may have significant intellectual subnormality.

The Child With Depressed Potential

For some years it has been recognized that factors other than intellectual subnormality affected achievement in the classroom. Concern in our schools today for the disadvantaged and

---

[3]Samuel A. Kirk, *Educating Exceptional Children.* Boston, Houghton Mifflin, 1962, pp. 85-86.
[4]Gunnar Dywab, Who are the mentally retarded? *Children,* 15:44, 1968.

culturally different children is placing increased emphasis on an understanding of these factors. Several decades ago these factors were considered by Featherstone in his delineation of the term *slow learners.*[5] He differentiated the limited educational achievement of the *constitutional slow learner* with subnormal intellectual capacity from the *functional slow learner.* The latter is often mistaken by teachers for a slow learner with limited potential because he is having difficulty achieving in the classroom. He may be making limited progress in acquiring the academic skills or he may be a behavior problem, but his limited achievements are caused by numerous other factors that serve to depress an individual's ability to learn. Such factors may be the lack of psychosocial stimulation from limited socioeconomic environment, inadequate hearing and vision, emotional problems in relationships with family and peers, malnutrition or poor general health. It is important to recognize that the situation is not necessarily permanent. Both educational programs and conditions affecting the child's physical, social, emotional and intellectual well-being can be improved.

The Child With A Learning Disability

A further compounding of the problem of identification of the *slow learner* has occurred with studies of children who do not come under the categories of the *constitutional* or *functional slow learner,* but whose classroom achievement may be similar. Johnson and Myklebust warn of the imperative need for proper identification of these children, "Often the child with a learning disability is labeled slow or lazy when in reality he is neither. These labels have an adverse effect on future learning, on self perception, and on feelings of personal worth."[6]

The research identifying learning-disability children indicates

---

[5]W. B. Featherstone, Teaching the slow learner. In Caswell, Hollis L. (Ed.):*Practical Suggestion for Teaching,* 2nd ed. New York, Teachers College, Columbia University, 1951, No. 1, pp. 10-11.

[6]Doris J. Johnson and Helmer R. Myklebust, *Learning Disabilities.* New York, Grune & Stratton, 1967, p. 49.

that their learning has been impaired in specific areas of verbal and/or nonverbal learning, but their *potential* for learning is categorized as normal or above. Thus, these learning disability children fall within the 90 and above IQ range in either the verbal or nonverbal areas. Total IQ is not used as the criterion for determining learning potential inasmuch as adequate intelligence, either verbal or nonverbal, may be obscured in cases where the total IQ falls below 90, but in which specific aspects of intelligence fall within the definition of adequate intelligence. The learning-disability child whose IQ falls below the normal range, and where a learning disability is present is considered to have a multiple involvement.

In learning-disability children there are deficits in verbal and/or nonverbal learning. There may be impairment of expressive, receptive or integrative functions. There is concern for deficits in the function of input and output, of sensory modalities and overloading, and of degree of impairment. The essential differences of the mentally retarded and the learning-disability child have been characterized as the following:

> One cannot deny that the neurology of learning has been disturbed in the mentally retarded, but the fundamental effect has been to reduce potential for learning in general. Though some retarded children have isolated *high* levels of function, the pattern is one of generalized inferiority; normal potential for learning is *not* assumed. In comparison, children with learning disabilities have isolated *low* levels of function. The pattern is one of generalized integrity of mental capacity; normal potential is assumed.[7]

Consequently, the learning disability child shows marked differences from the child with limited potential. There are both qualitative and quantitative differences. The learning disability child has more potential for learning. The means by which he learns are different.

While there may be some overlapping in the educational methods used with these three groups identified as *slow learners*,

---

[7]Doris J. Johnson and Helmer R. Myklebust, *Learning Disabilities*. New York, Grune & Stratton, 1967, p. 55.

there obviously must be differentiation in educational goals and approaches for these various groups. Correct identification of the factors causing *slowness in learning* is essential in teaching with the individual differences among children. The theories and practices presented in this text suggest an effective approach for teachers to use in working with the child most appropriately identified as the *constitutional slow learner*. However, it is recognized that the approach to learning through motor activity is also very appropriate in many situations for those children with learning problems caused by factors other than subnormal intellectual functioning.

LEARNING CHARACTERISTICS OF THE SLOW LEARNER

When considering educational processes that would provide a successful learning experience for children with limited intellectual potential, it is necessary to examine some of their basic characteristics of learning as found from numerous studies. *Slow learners* appear to follow the same patterns as those who have more adequate intellectual endowment in terms of the sequence of growth and development. The basic difference is the time schedule at which these children arrive at various levels of development. Theoretically, the child with an IQ of 80 develops intellectually at a rate only four-fifths that of the average child. The rate of development of these children is more closely correlated with their mental age than their chronological age.

In a summation of the research on the learning characteristics of the mentally retarded, Johnson emphasized some time ago that they learn in the same way as normal children. The studies indicate "remarkable agreement in the results, regardless of the environment or degree of intellectual deficit."[8]
Johnson concludes,

> Although the two groups (normal and mentally handicapped) may differ significantly on such developmental factors as life age, physical and motor development, or social

---

[8]C. Orville Johnson, Psychological characteristics of the mentally retarded. In Cruikshank, William M. (Ed.): *Psychology of Exceptional Children and Youth*, 2nd ed. Englewood Cliffs, Prentice-Hall, 1963, p. 457.

development, as long as they are equated for intellectual developmental levels, experiences, and previous learnings to ensure equal readiness, they should have similar patterns of learning, require the same amounts of practice, and retain equal amount of material learned.[9]

Differences have been found in comparison of the learning processes in arithmetic and reading of the mentally retarded and normal children. However, according to Johnson, these differences are not attributable to *ability* to learn but to the influence of instructional procedures. Included among the factors affecting the learning process are the value systems of the individual and his own concept of self as a learner. These two factors must be recognized as particularly important. The reason for this is that there are so many negative psychosocial factors operating within the life space of large percentages of the mentally retarded who can maintain themselves only in a low socioeconomic environment.

Kirk's studies relating to the effect of preschool education on the development of educable mentally retarded children have shown that school experience can make a difference on rate of development. He has indicated that, "It would appear that although the upper limits of development for an individual are genetically or organically determined, the functional level or rate of development may be accelerated or depressed within the limits set by the organism. Somatopsychological factors and the cultural milieu (including schooling) are capable of influencing the functional level within these limits.[10]

PRINCIPLES OF LEARNING FOR SLOW LEARNERS APPLIED TO MOTOR ACTIVITY

In providing appropriate learning experiences for slow learners, it is essential to help them be successful by structuring

[9]C. Orville Johnson, Psychological characteristics of the mentally retarded. In Cruikshank, William M. (Ed.): *Psychology of Exceptional Children and Youth,* 2nd ed. Englewood Cliffs, Prentice-Hall, 1963, p. 461.
[10]Samuel A. Kirk, Educating Exceptional Children. Boston, Houghton Mifflin, 1962, pp. 100-101.

activities to reflect the best principles of learning. Various individuals have suggested certain principles of learning that are applicable to slow learners. A list of such principles which seems useful for our purpose is one set forth by Kirk.[11] The principles are listed as follows with implications for learning through motor activity suggested by the present author.

1. Progress is from the known to the unknown, using concrete materials to foster understanding of more abstract facts.

Implication: Use of motor activity helps children act out, and see and feel the concepts being developed, thus it becomes a part of their *physical reality*.

2. The child is helped to transfer known abilities from one situation to another rather than being expected to make generalizations spontaneously.

Implication: Movement-oriented experiences enable children to work out the relationship of one situation with another and to make appropriate transfer of skills and generalizations easily.

3. The teacher may use many repetitions in a variety of experiences.

Implication: Motor activities such as active games, rhythmic activities and stunts provide a pleasurable, highly motivating means for necessary repetition which is not· objectionable to children.

4. Learning is stimulated through exciting situations.

Implication: Personal involvement, high interest and motivation are concomitant with learning through motor activity.

5. Inhibitions are avoided by presenting one idea at a time and presenting learning situations by sequential steps.

Implication: The structure of a motor activity such as an active game in itself implies logical ordering of ideas that are dramatized through physical movement.

6. Learning is reinforced through using a variety of sensory modalities — visual, vocal, auditory, kinesthetic.

Implication: Motor learning heightens the learning act when integrated with verbal learning experiences.

Such guidelines emphasize the need for total involvement of

---

[11]Samuel A. Kirk, Educating Exceptional Children. Boston, Houghton Mifflin, 1962, pp. 121.

the learner, for using the concrete experience to develop an abstract concept, and for providing for continuity and transference of one learning experience to another. A good many years ago Featherstone also stressed the need for working with the concrete, "One of the chief reasons for emphasizing activities based upon very concrete and tangible or objective things rather than upon predominantly verbal or abstract things is that such activities usually permit more demonstrating, constructing, picturing, and dramatizing as means of communicating ideas."[12]

Such techniques are more likely to ensure successful learning for all children, regardless of intellectual potential; for slow learners they are essential. The use of motor activity to develop abstract concepts in the various curriculum areas is therefore sound methodology for all learners and particularly appropriate for the slow learner. The representative examples that follow point this up more clearly.

Case 1

In using the game STRADDLE BALL ROLL described in the introductory chapter with a heterogeneous group of fourth grade children to develop the concept, *electricity travels along a pathway and needs a complete circuit over which to travel,* the following was observed.

The children quickly made the analogy themselves after noticing how interference in the path of the ball caused it to go out of bounds and stop the game. In a similar manner, blockage of an electric current would break the circuit and stop the flow of electricity.

An experiment with wired batteries and a bell had also been used in connection with the development of this concept. Three of the slower learning children reported that they understood this better after they had played Straddle Ball Roll because they could actually *see* the electric current, which in this case was the ball.

---

[12]W. B. Featherstone, Teaching the slow learner. In Caswell, Hollis L. (Ed.): Practical Suggestion for Teaching, 2nd ed. New York, Teachers College, Columbia University, 1951, No. 1, pp. 10-11.

Case 2

In a special education class the teacher attempted to develop the concept of *self body image* through an active game called BUSY BEE. In this game the children are in pairs facing each other and dispersed around the activity area. One child who is the *caller* is in the center of the area. He makes calls such as *shoulder to shoulder, toe to toe,* or *hand to hand.* (In the early stages of the game it was necessary for the teacher to do the calling.) As the calls are made, the paired children go through the appropriate motions with their partners. After a few calls the caller will shout, "Busy Bee!" This is the signal for every child to get a new partner, including the caller. The child who does not get a partner can become the new caller.

As the children played the game, the teacher made them aware of the location of various parts of their body in order to develop the concept of full body image.

Before the game was played, the children were asked to draw a picture of themselves. Many did not know how to begin, and others omitted some of the major limbs in their drawings. After playing Busy Bee, the children were again asked to draw a picture of themselves. This time they were more successful. All of the drawings had bodies, heads, arms and legs. Some of them had hands, feet, eyes and ears. A few even had teeth and hair.

Case 3

This illustration involved a class of fourteen children, nine years, two months to twelve years, two months of age, with an IQ range from 60 to 85. Two examples of motor activities used with this class follow.

In the first activity the teacher was attempting to develop a better understanding of addition facts. The activity used for this purpose was EXCHANGE NUMBERS. Seven 6 by 8-inch index cards are used with a number from six to twelve on one side of each. On the other side are written the combinations which, when added together, give the sum of the number on the opposite side. For example, if the number on one side were twelve, then the combinations on the other side would be

6	7	8	9	10	11	12
6	5	4	3	2	1	0

A duplicate of these cards is made. Each pupil is given a card, with two pupils having identical cards. The leader stands in front of the class and calls out two numbers. The pupils having the sum of these two numbers try to exchange places before being tagged by the leader. After playing the game for a time, a new leader can be selected, or the person tagged may become the leader.

The pupils made the cards during the regular arithmetic class and were told that they were to be used later during a play period in a new game. Numbers from six to twelve were given to the pupils, with two pupils having the same number. The class was paired off, with the two pupils who had the same number being together. The pairs went to the chalkboard to work out the combinations which, when added together, gave the sum of their respective numbers. Then they checked their answers for accuracy on the abacus, with the teacher giving guidance as needed. They returned to their desks to make the cards. Each pupil made one card.

The game was explained and played during the play period which, because of rain, had to take place in the classroom. The leader called two numbers, and the two pupils having the sum of the two numbers stood and attempted to change seats before being tagged. The pupil tagged became *It*. One of the problems that arose in the game was that sometimes one child would understand the combination before the other. He would have no place to run to and would be tagged because the other child did not move from his seat. To correct this, it was decided that the runner could stand and touch the back of his chair and be safe until he other person stood up. The leader had to stay in front of the room until someone left his seat.

In evaluating this activity, it was observed that the preparation for the activity gave experience in addition and writing numbers, and that the children were more motivated to do this when they found they were going to use the cards in a game. The pupils saw a purpose in learning the addition facts and in checking for accuracy as well as making legible figures. They also had a better understanding of *pairs* and *exchange*. The fact that a pleasurable use for the addition facts was created was valuable. The pupils were aware that listening was important, that it was necessary to run and dodge quickly, and that they had to be careful to avoid running into each other. They enjoyed the activity very much and asked to play the game during indoor recess.

The second example with this class was concerned with recognition of beginning sounds. The activity used for this purpose was a version of STEAL THE BACON. The class was divided into two teams of seven each and stood ten feet apart, facing each other. The members of both teams were given the letter *b, c, d, h, m, n* and *p* as in the following diagram because the class had been having difficulty with the beginning consonants.

b		*p*
c		*n*
d		*m*
h	beanbag	*h*
m	(bacon)	*d*
n		*c*
p		*b*

The teacher called out a word such as *ball,* and the two pupils having the letter *b* ran out to grab the beanbag. If the player got the beanbag back to his line, he scored two points for his team. If his opponent tagged him before he got back, the other team scored one point. The game ended when each letter had been called. After the scores were totaled, the game was repeated at the request of the children. When the game was continued, the children were identified with different letters.

In evaluating this activity, the children pointed out that listening was important in order to understand the letter called. This was particularly necessary to distinguish the sounds of *b* and *d* and *m* and *n*. It was also necessary to run and dodge rapidly in order to achieve the goal. They also mentioned that they had to know about addition in order to keep score.

The intent of the first four chapters of the text has been to present a generalized picture of the potential for learning through motor activity. The final five chapters focus upon the use of motor activity for learning in the specific curriculum areas of reading, mathematics, science, social studies and health and safety.

CHAPTER FIVE.

LEARNING TO READ
THROUGH MOTOR ACTIVITY

As far back as the late seventeenth century Fénelon (1651-1715) is reputed to have said, "I have seen certain children who have learned to read while playing."[1] If one were the least bit given to rationalization, it could be speculated that this statement might well have been the first indication that there is a high level of compatibility between reading and motor activity, and a forerunner to some beliefs of the current day.

In any event, in modern times the sensorimotor aspects of the real experience, the bringing of physical reality to the printed word and page through proprioception are cited over and over again in the literature as facilitating and enhancing perception and cognition. In addition, the naturalness of the physically-oriented activity for beginning and early readers is recognized. This author recognizes that the reading act ultimately emphasizes the representational nature of word symbols, and that the higher levels of cognition are abstract. However, it is not an either-or situation. There is general agreement that the physical reality of concrete experience aids comprehension. There is evidence that there is need for increased emphasis upon the use of the physical reality of the child in his learning-to-read efforts.

The subsequent discussions in this chapter will outline several suggestions and recommendations utilizing motor activities that have been found effective in skill development and establishing interest and positive attitudes toward reading.

MOTOR-ORIENTED READING CONTENT

Basic facts about the nature of human beings serve educators

---

[1] George Ellsworth Johnson, *Education by Plays and Games*. Boston, Ginn and Company, 1907, p. 31.

today as principles of learning. One of these principles, *desirable learning takes place when the child has his own purposeful goals to guide his learning activities,* serves as the basis for developing motor-oriented reading content material.

One of the early and perhaps the first attempt to prepare motor-oriented reading content as conceived here is the work of the present author and one of his associates.[2] This original work involved a detailed study of reactions of six-to-eight-year-old children when independent reading material is oriented to active game participation. This experiment was initiated on the premise of relating reading content for children to their natural urge to play.

The original study utilizing active games written with a story setting has been described in *Chapter Three.* From this study additional stories were developed and published as the *Read and Play Series.*[3] This series consists of six books in which there are 131 stories. Set One of the series is for first grade and Set Two is for second grade. Each set consists of three books. The stories in the first two books in each set are written around active games or stunt settings. The third book in each set is written around a rhythmic or dance setting.

This carefully developed material, in terms of readability, the reading values and literary merit of the stories, utilizes children's natural affinity for motor-oriented play as the motivation for their reading. This unique reading content calls for active responses to the reading task, the task being one that involves learning to play an active game or to perform physically-oriented stunts or rhythms. Such tasks bring a physical reality to printed word symbols.

Motor-oriented reading content material, while enriching and extending the child's experiences, reinforces his general ability to read through his reading independently and "on his own." A child or group of children may read a story individually, in buddy

---

[2]James H. Humphrey and Virginia D. Moore, Improving reading through physical education. *Education* (The Reading Issue), May, 1960, p. 559.

[3]James H. Humphrey and Virginia D. Moore, *Read and Play Series.* London, Frederick Muller, Ltd., Ludgate House, 1965.

teams or as a group with the teacher providing individual help with words when needed. After reading the story the child or children play the game or perform the stunt or rhythmic activity. They may then reread the story and discuss how they might improve upon their first attempt at carrying out the motor-oriented task. With this procedure the child is able to develop cognitive processing skills through the physical reality of the activity involved. The child is therefore provided opportunities to practice and maintain skills necessary for meaningful reading.

A further dimension of the stories such as the read and play approach is the unique purpose-setting and problem-solving nature inherent in the reading activities of the stories. The child is reading to find out how to do something — play a game or do a stunt. The child is using all his skills in reading to solve the problem of performing the task described in the story. Both purpose-setting and problem-solving have been identified as essential to the higher cognitive processes in mature reading. Such reading activities as the read and play approach can provide children their first opportunities to exercise these skills with physically real experiences.

Furthermore, this approach enables the teacher to assess the child's vocabulary development and how well comprehension skills are being practiced because the children actually demonstrate their understanding of what they read. Thus, the teacher can observe by their actions the children's comprehension of the material. This relates closely with the use of motor-oriented learning activities as a means of diagnosing skills in reading discussed later in this chapter.

Introducing the Material

After the prepared stories have been made available for the classroom library the teacher may introduce several stories by reading them to the children, then having the children play the game or demonstrate the stunt or rhythm. Stories developing each type of physical activity should be selected so children will understand how the stories provide details they can use to figure how to perform a stunt or rhythmic activity or to play a game.

Sample stories should also be selected to demonstrate that some stories can be acted out by an individual child and that some require several children to participate in the stunt or game. This latter aspect of the motor-oriented reading content material utilizes another basic principle of learning — *desirable learning takes place when the child is given the opportunity to share cooperatively in learning experiences with his classmates* under the guidance, but not the control of the teacher. The point to be emphasized here is that although learning may be an individual matter, it is likely to take place best in a group. This is to say that children learn individually, but that socialization should be retained. Moreover, sharing in group activities is an important essential in educating for democracy.

After the teacher reads a sample story the children are asked to carry out the activity. As the children carry out the activity the teacher accepts their efforts. The teacher may provide guidance *only* to the extent it is necessary to help the children identify problems and provide opportunity for them to exercise judgment in solving them and obtaining their goal, that of playing the game or performing the stunt or rhythm. Parts of the story might be reread by the teacher if the children have difficulty in understanding how to carry out the activity. The children might be encouraged to discuss ways they could help themselves remember the details of the story, e.g. by pretending they are *George Giraffe* or that they were really playing the game, they might take more time and read more carefully to recall details better.

Independent Reading and Follow-Up Play Activities

After such an introduction to the prepared stories, the children should be encouraged to read them "on their own." The teacher and children might plan several procedures for using the stories. Such activities might include:

1. A group of children may select and read a story for a physical education activity.

2. Individual children may select stories involving the individual stunts for a physical education period.

3. After reading one of the Read and Play books an individual child may elect to act out his favorite stunt story before a group of children. (The children might be asked who or what the story describes.)

4. After reading one of the stories an individual might get several other children to read the story and participate in playing the game.

5. Children might use a buddy system for reading and acting out stories.

6. Children might write and illustrate similar-type stories for other children to read and act out.

The following is a specific suggestion for procedures that might be utilized in working with the basic types of stories that appear in the *Read and Play Series.* In this situation during which the children are taking turns acting out their favorite stunt story the teacher might direct the following discussion after a child's presentation of *George Giraffe.*[4]

George Giraffe

There is a tall animal in a far away land.
He has a long neck.
His name is George Giraffe.
You could look like him if you did this.
Place your arms high over your head.
Put your hands together.
Point them to the front.
This will be his neck and head.
Now walk like George Giraffe.
This is how.
Stand on your toes.
Walk with your legs straight.

Could you walk so you would look like George Giraffe?
TEACHER: Wasn't that interesting the way Johnny showed us

---

[4]James H. Humphrey and Virginia D. Moore, Read and Play Series. London, Frederick Muller, Ltd., Ludgate House, Set 1, Book 1, p. 30.

how George Giraffe looked? (Children) What do you think George Giraffe looked like from what Johnny did? (Children) What did Johnny do to look like George Giraffe? What did Johnny do to have a long neck like George Giraffe? (Children) Can someone else make a long neck? (Children demonstrate.) Oh, you are *all* very good at making long necks. Particularly Jimmy. How did Johnny walk to be like George Giraffe? Can someone show me? (Children demonstrate.) What do you have to do to walk like a giraffe? (Children) Is it easy to pretend to be a giraffe? Let's try it and find out. (All children demonstrate.) Did you feel awkward? (Children) We often say that giraffes look ungainly or awkward. Do you think these are good words to describe a giraffe? (Children) Can you think of other words we might use to describe a giraffe? (Children) Can you think of other animals that also look awkward or ungainly? (Children) That was good, Johnny. You really showed us how to look like a giraffe. You must have read the story very carefully. Bobby, you said you also had read the story about George Giraffe. Why do I say "Johnny must have read very carefully?" (Bobby) That's right. It is important to use all the information the story gives us to help you pretend to be something. That was fun, wasn't it? (Children) All right. Now Mary is going to tell us about her story. But this time we are going to do it differently. This time Mary is *not* going to tell us the name of her story or what she is pretending to be. We will have to guess *who* or *what* she is. (In this manner the group continues to share, discuss, act out and evaluate the stories the children present.)

Stories Developed by the Teacher

Motor-oriented content stories can be developed by the teacher. This has been successfully done by teachers who have produced amazingly creative stories using games, stunts and rhythms. Teachers have also involved children in such projects as creative writing experiences. In writing such stories using a motor-activity setting there are several guidelines that the teacher should keep in mind.

In general the new word load should be kept relatively low. There should be as much repetition of these words as possible and appropriate. Sentence length and lack of complexity in sentences should be considered in keeping the level of difficulty of material within the independent reading levels of children. There are numerous readability formulas that can be utilized. For primary-level stories Spache's Readability Formula[5] and MaGinnis' revision of Fry's Readability Graph[6] are best suited. For upper-level stories Fry's Readability Graph is useful.

Consideration must also be given to the reading values and literary merits of the story. Using a character or characters in a story setting helps to develop interest. The activity to be used in the story should *not* be readily identifiable. When children identify an activity early in the story there can be resulting minimum attention on the part of the reader to get the necessary details in order to play the game or perform the stunt or rhythmic activity. In developing an activity story, therefore, it is important that the nature of the activity and procedures for it unfold gradually.

In developing a story, the equipment, playing area and procedures should be clearly described. Basic motor skills that can be utilized in stunt and rhythmic activities as well as for games include *locomotor skills* (walking, running, leaping, jumping, hopping, skipping, galloping and sliding); *throwing and striking skills; catching* and *axial movements* such as twisting, turning and stretching.

When writing about games they should be at the developmental level of children. At the primary level games should involve a few simple rules and, in some cases, elementary strategies. Games that involve chasing and fleeing, tag and one small group against another, as well as those involving fundamental skills mentioned above are suggested. The games should be simple enough to be easy to learn, and they should capitalize upon the imitative and dramatic interests which are typical of this age. (This applies to stunt and rhythmic stories as well.) Children at the upper elementary level retain an interest in

---

[5]George D. Spache, *Good Books for Poor Readers*, Champaign, Garrard Publishing C., 1966. (The Spache Readability Formula was used with the *Read and Play Series*.)
[6]George H. MaGinnis, The readability graph and informal reading inventories. *The Reading Teacher*, March, 1969.

some of the games they played at the primary level, and some of them can be extended and made more difficult to meet the needs and interests of these older children. In addition, games may now be introduced which call for greater bodily control; finer coordination of hands, eyes and feet; and more strength.

In summary, motor-oriented reading content provides variety to the reading program. High interest and motivation are the results of purposeful reading and bringing words into physical reality by playing a game, performing a stunt or responding to a rhythm.

LEARNING TO READ THROUGH CREATIVE MOVEMENT — THE AMAV SEQUENCE

There appears to be rather general agreement on the intellectual needs of children. Some of these include (1) a need for challenging experiences at their own level, (2) a need for intellectually successful and satisfying experiences, (3) a need for the opportunity to solve problems, and (4) a need for opportunity to participate in creative experiences instead of always having to conform.[7]

For many years, creativity and giving the child an opportunity to be creative have been widely discussed. When a term is used so often and, in fact, in so many different frames of reference, it becomes difficult to understand its meaning. For this reason and for the author's purposes here, there is a need to identify the meaning of the term as it pertains to the present discussion. In this discussion creativity will be used in terms of giving a child his own freedom to respond to perceived situations. This, of course, should be done with various degrees of teacher guidance since children vary in their ability to be creative. This is particularly true in the early stages of the more inhibited children.

This line of thought is compatible with a very important principle of learning — *desirable learning takes place when the child is free to create his own responses in the situation he faces.*[8]

---

[7]James H. Humphrey, *Child Learning Through Elementary School Physical Education*, 2nd ed. Dubuque, Wm. C. Brown Publishers, 1974, p. 22-24.
[8]James H. Humphrey, Child Learning Through Elementary School Physical Eduation, 2nd ed. Dubuque, Wm. C. Brown, Publishers, 1974, p 68.

This principle indicates that problem-solving is the way of human learning and that the child will learn largely only through direct or indirect experience. This implies that the teacher should provide every opportunity for children to utilize judgment in the various perceived situations that arise. It takes the utmost skill on the part of the teacher to know when to "step in and teach," and when to remain in the background so that further learning may take place. When the child is free to create his own responses in the situation he faces, individual differences must obviously be taken into consideration.

It is interesting to note that a great deal is heard about the so-called *creative method* or the *problem-solving method*. Actually, these might not be methods at all, but rather applications of the previously stated valid principle of learning. Creativity and problem-solving should not be isolated as specific methods, but should be involved in all types of methods.

One of the utmost concerns to educators is the problem of how to provide for creative expression so that a child may develop his potentialities fully. In fact, researchers are only beginning to understand the power of the individual as perhaps a most dynamic force in the world today. It is in this frame of reference that creativity should come clearly into focus because many of the problems in our society can be solved only through creative thinking.

Creative experience involves self-expression. It is concerned with the need to experiment, to express original ideas, to think and to react. Children are naturally creative — they imagine, they pretend, they are uninhibited. They are not only original, but actually ingenious in their thoughts and actions. Indeed, creativity is a characteristic inherent to some degree in the lives of practically all children. Some children create as a natural form of expression without adult stimulation while others may need varying amounts of teacher guidance and encouragement. School need not stifle the creative nature within children, yet it often does. Particularly in language arts we find teachers inhibiting the child's freedom of response. In the apparent necessity for every child to work quietly in his seat, creativity may be inhibited.

There is a variety of media for creative expression (art, music and writing) which are considered the traditional approaches to creative expression. A vital means of creative expression, one too often overlooked, is movement. Movement utilizes the body as the instrument of expression. For the young child, the most natural form of creative expression is movement. Children have a natural inclination for movement, and they use this medium as the basic form of creative expression. Movement is the child's universal language, a most important form of communication and a most meaningful way of learning.

A procedure for learning to read through creative movement, termed the *AMAV Technique,* was developed by the author with the assistance of two collaborators in the reading field. This original work consists of four stories on two long-play records or cassettes, a teacher's manual and sets of eight booklets of the stories, the source of which is:

> Robert M. Wilson, James H. Humphrey and Dorothy D. Sullivan, *Teaching Reading Through Creative Movement.* The AMAV Technique, Kimbo Educational, Deal, New Jersey, 1969.

The AMAV Technique involves a learning sequence of *auditory input* to *movement* to *auditory-visual input* as depicted in the following diagram.

*A*uditory ——→ Movement ——→ *A*uditory ——→ *V*isual

Essentially the AMAV Technique is a procedure for working through creative movement to develop comprehension, first in listening, and then in reading. The A ——→ M aspect of AMAV is a directed listening-thinking activity. Children first receive the thoughts and feelings expressed in a story through the auditory sense by listening to a recorded story. Following this they engage in movement experiences which are inherent in the story, and thereby demonstrate their understanding of and reaction to the story. By engaging in the movement, the development of comprehension becomes a part of the child's physical reality.

After the creative movement experience in the directed listening-thinking activity the children move to the final aspect of the AMAV Technique (A-V), a combination of auditory and visual experience by listening to the story and reading along in the story booklet. In this manner comprehension is brought to the reading experience.

Although the comprehension skills for listening and reading are the same, the sensory input is different — that is listening is dependent upon the auditory sense, and reading is dependent upon the visual sense. The sequence of listening to reading is a natural one. However, bridging the gap to the point of handling the verbal symbols required in reading poses various problems for many children. One of the outstanding features of the AMAV Technique is that the movement experience helps to serve as a bridge between listening and reading by providing direct purposeful experience for the child through creative movement after listening to the story.

Another version of the AMAV Technique where the teacher provides the auditory input by reading shorter stories to the children is found in the following source:

> James H. Humphrey, *Learning to Listen and Read Through Movement*. Deal, Kimbo Educational, 1974.

(This book contains over sixty stories about games, stunts and rhythms with complete instructions for use with listening and reading skills.)

It is possible for teachers to prepare their own materials to teach children to read through creative movement using the AMAV Technique. Although such a procedure would not likely be so detailed as the original published work and is somewhat of a painstaking task, it can provide an interesting activity for a creative teacher. Preparing such materials can also be creative projects for older children. Remedial readers can help to prepare such materials for younger children.

DIAGNOSIS THROUGH MOTOR ACTIVITY

Diagnostic teaching is today's byword as school systems address their attention to meeting the individual needs of children. This applies particularly to reading instruction through the nationwide "Right to Read" program.

Over the years the term *diagnosis* has generally been thought of as a more formal out-of-classroom procedure for those children the teacher identifies as having difficulties in their attempts to learn to read. Occasionally diagnosis is requested for those children whom teachers consider as not working up to their potential. But today, more and more specialists in reading are recognizing that in most cases classroom diagnosis can provide adequate information about reading skill strengths and needs of children to help the classroom teacher make appropriate adjustments in instruction. Such adjustments involve focus on specific skills, levels of material and methods of instruction.

Classroom diagnosis has been directed to assessing the skill strengths and needs of children, either prior to or after instruction. Traditional measures have been standardized tests (usually survey in nature), informal inventories or teacher-made tests. In recent years the value of teacher observations of children during different types of reading situations has been recognized as essential to supplement information received from the traditional measures. Such observations are followed by recording and analyzing their reading performances.

The procedure of observing, recording and analyzing a child's performance during the learning activity has come to be recognized as perhaps a more reliable assessment of his skills development. Such procedures have become the framework for diagnostic teaching. Bond has described diagnostic teaching as being "based on an understanding of the *reading* strengths and needs of each child. These knowledges must be used to modify instructional procedures so that teaching, adjusted to the changing needs of children, can be maintained. Such teaching is based on continuous diagnosis of the skill development of each child."[9] It is at this point that the use of motor activities can play a unique role in diagnosis.

One of the many problems inherent in testing situations is the effect of a child's apprehension on his performance of the task involved. Basic principles of clinical diagnosis in reading have

[9]Guy L. Bond, Diagnostic teaching in the classroom. DeBoer, Dorothy L. (Ed.): *Reading Diagnosis and Evaluation*. Newark, Delaware, International Reading Association, 1970, pp. 130-131.

alluded to this problem by emphasizing the importance of establishing rapport with the child, starting the testing with less threatening types of tasks, and stopping at the first frustration level before complete discouragement disintegrates the testing situation. Teachers using such classroom diagnostic measures as mentioned often voice a concern relating to this apprehension on the part of children. They realize that the child must be put at ease as to the nature and the reason for testing. Paper-and-pencil tests throughout the grades, along with the aptitude tests and college entrance examinations, have resulted in adult aversion of test-taking to the point of significant blocking of what might well be a usual performance level of an individual when not under stress.

Diagnostic teaching techniques employing observation, recording and analysis of children's performance in day-to-day reading situations has become a significant trend in assessment. Obtaining daily feedback is a key to structuring appropriate day-to-day learning activities because they are based on the real reading performance of the child. It is a better *reading* of where the child is in his skills development. Therefore, in diagnostic teaching, teachers are using such techniques as coding errors made by children while oral reading to prove points in the discussion of the material they are reading for a directed reading-thinking activity. In this way the teacher has information about the children's sight vocabulary, word attack application to unfamiliar words in context reading, and comprehension skills.

The every-pupil-response technique is used by the teacher as a diagnostic teaching procedure in many types of situations. With the technique calling for each child in a group to respond to a question or problem by holding up an answer card or signaling with a finger response a choice of answers, the teacher is able to check the performance of all the children. The teacher can observe each child's understanding and interpretation of the material and his application of a specific skill to new words as in the case of reading. This technique not only provides information about each child's skills development within a group activity, but it also involves each child consistently throughout the learning and application of skills. This aspect of maximum involvement of each child within a group activity is particularly inherent in motor activities. An example of this is the game MATCH CATS which is described later in the chapter.

Teachers are also using games as a means of assessing the level of mastery of skills to determine whether further instructional activities need to be planned. Such reading games have been essentially *passive* in nature rather than *active*. The techniques as described for diagnostic teaching have served the teacher well in efforts to develop a reading program that meets the individual needs of all children.

It is interesting to note that these diagnostic techniques are geared to observing an individual child's performance within group learning activities. Teachers employing these techniques have reported they are better able to plan further activities for children to meet their individual needs through subgrouping children for additional learning experiences. As a result, the individualizing of instruction, a major objective of schools, becomes a reality.

Motor Activities as a Diagnostic Teaching Technique

As previously mentioned, the unique role of motor activities in classroom diagnosis becomes evident when active games as a diagnostic teaching technique are discussed. By adding the dimension of motor involvement to game activities, the use of children's naturally physically-oriented world becomes a positive factor operating to facilitate further interest as well as more involvement in attending to the learning task. Many children tend to lose their apprehension of an intellectual task when it is buried in the context of a motor activity.

In particular, disabled readers will often perform tasks such as auditory and visual discrimination while playing a game when they would be saying "I can't do it" in more traditional learning activities. *Active* games tend to draw out the reluctant learner even more than *passive* games. Observation of children with severe reading problems, whose discouragement and frustration initially hampers their willingness to even participate, has shown their natural affinity for physical activity to be a more accurate starting point for assessment of their skill strengths, needs and remediation.

The total physical involvement of such children in motor activities related to reading appears to act as a means for releasing the emotional blockage that inhibits any attempt to perform the intellectual reading tasks involved. Once these children participate successfully in such activities, because of the strengthening of input through their physical world, the process of building more positive attitudes toward reading and the feeling that they can learn are begun. Needless to say, once the teacher has observed a higher-level performance of children in this setting, it is important to help the children recognize that they were able to, and did, perform the skill involved. Such children need to be shown they *can* and *have* mastered a skill with specific evidence that they have learned.

While the initial focus of motor activities has been on *active* games as useful diagnostic tools, motor-oriented reading content materials and creative movement activities are also conducive to diagnosis. Once again the teacher is able to observe a child demonstrating a level of skills development from the reading tasks utilized in the activity in a natural setting.

Four important factors in motor activities that the teacher utilizes to determine whether further learning experiences are necessary for skill mastery are (1) the type of sensory input or modality involved in the reading task inherent in the motor activity, (2) the accuracy of the child's responses in the reading task, (3) the reaction time of children performing that reading task, and (4) the self-evaluation of the child of his performance.

Sound instructional programs have always been oriented toward a specific skill. The impact of establishing behaviorally-stated goals as objectives for instruction has helped teachers to move beyond such lesson plan goals as "learning word attack skills" to "being able to identify by name the initial letter of a word given orally," or "being able to give orally another word that begins with the same sound as a word presented visually." In the latter lesson objectives, both input and output modality are clearly stated so that a teacher observing such activities can analyze children's performances in regard to sensory modality both for input and output production. Such information helps the teacher to identify those children who consistently give evidence of significant differences in performance when lesson input is basically auditory or visual. Such information helps the teacher to adapt instruction accordingly, and thereby assures more meaningful and more successful learning-to-read experiences. Different modalities are used in different games, e.g. the signal to start the game may involve auditory input such as "Hill Dill run over the hill" in the game of HILL DILL. In others, visual input such as displaying a certain color is the signal to start the game.

The second factor in motor activities which a teacher utilizes is the accuracy of children's responses to the reading tasks inherent in the activity. It can be observed that those children who use the specific skill with at least 90 percent accuracy in their responses represent skill mastery at the independent level. Any lower percentage of accuracy would indicate additional experiences are necessary.

The third factor relating to the reaction time of children's performance during motor activities helps the teacher identify the ease and comfort of children in performing a specific task. Reaction time in the present text refers to the amount of time it takes for the onset of a response of a person after receiving a stimulus. By observing the quickness of a child's response to the reading task inherent in the motor activity, the teacher can assess the degree of ease as well as the accuracy of the child's responses. While percentage of accuracy is a useful and necessary tool in determining when a child reaches the point of skill mastery, the ease and comfort of the child during the reading task is also a significant factor. Skill mastery implies operation at an automatic level independently.

Of particular concern in consideration of reaction time are those children who have a disability in processing the sensory input with a resulting delay in reaction to the question or task presented. Such impairment can effect auditory, visual or feeling input. This may be related to the first factor in the use of motor activities as a diagnostic tool in which the teacher observes children's performances in terms of modality used. In the game CALL AND CATCH described later, the teacher can adjust the timing by momentarily holding the ball before throwing it into the air. In the case of reaction time there may simply be a lesser degree of impairment resulting only in more reaction time necessary to perform the task. The teacher must be aware that children may have this type of disability and attempt to recognize those children who consistently need additional time to respond to the task. It is important to adjust to the needs of such children rather than categorize their delay in responding as being the result of disinterest or uncooperativeness. Motor activities can easily be adapted to such children.

The fourth factor is that of self-evaluation by the children themselves. Children should be encouraged not only to react to the activity itself, but also to assess how they did and what they might do to improve their performances of the reading skill involved. It might be a case of looking more carefully at the word, picture or design cards used in the game. In such pleasurable activities children appear more willing to examine their performances in the learning tasks involved, and to examine them quite realistically.

The uniqueness of motor activities, therefore, as another means of classroom diagnosis, is that such activities tend to remove the apprehension of testing procedures and can demonstrate a level of skills development that is possibly more consistent with day-to-day performance. Such performance of the reading skill involved in the motor activity might even appear higher than when the children are engaged in more traditional reading activities. This higher level performance should be taken as a more accurate assessment of children's potential level of performance when they are operating under optimum conditions of learning.

Diagnosis of Reading Readiness Skills

Reading readiness skills are a complex cluster of basic skills including (1) language development in which the child learns to transform *his experience* with *his environment* into language symbols through listening, oral language facility and a meaningful vocabulary; (2) the skills relating to the mechanics of reading such as left-to-right orientation, auditory and visual discrimination, and recognition of letter names and sounds; and (3) the cognitive processes of comparing, classifying, ordering, interpreting, summarizing and imagining.

Likewise, sensorimotor skills provide a foundation for these basic skills by sharpening the senses and developing motor skills involving spatial, form and time concepts. The following outline identifies some concepts which can be developed through direct body movement:

1. Body Image (body parts, relating body and body parts to the environment, movement with body parts, usage of body parts)
2. Space and Direction (children point, move to objects)
3. Balance
4. Basic Body Movements (various locomotor skills)
5. Eye-Hand Coordination (ball bouncing, bean bag or ring toss)
6. Eye-Foot Coordination (propelling ball with feet)
7. Form Perception
8. Rhythm
9. Large Muscle Activity
10. Fine Muscle Activity (coordination and fine eye muscular movement)

These skills are extremely important to the establishment of a sound foundation for the beginning-to-read experiences of children. Not only can the reading readiness program, structured for the development of these skills, be facilitated through motor activities, but diagnosis of progress in skills development can be obtained by teacher observation and children's self-evaluation from the motor activities. Such physically-oriented activities as chasing and fleeing games, games of circle formation, stationary relays, rhythmic activities such as singing games, and creative rhythms can be utilized effectively to provide meaningful and satisfying learning activities in the reading readiness program. The following activities are described to indicate the variety of possibilities that may be employed in the development and assessment of readiness skills.

Language Development

In such activities as the following, concept formation is

translated into meaningful vocabulary.

Concept: Classification

Activity: Pet Store

One fairly large pet store is marked off at one end of the activity area and a home at the other end. At the side is a cage. In the center of the playing area stands the pet store owner. All the children stand in the pet store and are given a picture of one kind of pet, for example, bird, fish, dog. There should be about two or three pictures of each kind of pet. The pet store owner calls, fish, or any of the other pets in the game. The children who have pictures of fish must try to run from the pet store to their new home without being caught or tagged by the owner. If they are caught, they must go to the cage and wait for the next call. The game continues until all the pets have tried to get to their new home. Kinds of pets can be changed frequently.

Suggested Use: By grouping themselves according to the animal pictures, children are able to practice classifying things that swim, things that fly and so forth. At the end of the game the class can count how many fish, dogs and so forth were caught. All the fish, bird, dogs and so forth can then form their own line to *swim, fly* or *run* back to the pet store where new pictures can be given to the children for another game.

Concept: Vocabulary Meaning — Action Words

Activity: What to Play

The children may stand beside their desks. One of the children is selected to be the leader. While that child is coming to the front of the room to lead, the rest of the class begins to sing, to the tune of "Mary Had a Little Lamb,"

> Mary tell us what to play,
> What to play, what to play,
> Mary tell us what to play,
> Tell us what to play.

The leader then says, "Let's play we're fishes," or "Let's wash dishes." The leader then performs some action that the other children have to imitate. On a signal the children stop, and a new leader is selected.

Suggested Use: This activity gives children an opportunity to act out meanings of words. It helps them to recognize that spoken words represent actions of people as well as things that can be touched.

Concept: Vocabulary Meaning — Left and Right

Activity: Changing Seats

Enough chairs for each child in the group are placed side by side in about four or five rows. The children sit alert, ready to move either way. The teacher calls, "Change right!" and each child moves into the seat to his right. When the teacher calls, "Change left!" each child moves left. The child at the end of the row who does not have a seat to move to must run to the other end of his row and sit in the vacant seat there. The teacher can bring excitement to the game by the quickness of calls or unexpectedness by calling the same direction several times in succession. After each call the first row of children who all find seats may score a point for that row.

Suggested Use: This type of activity makes children more aware of the necessity of differentiating left from right. At the beginning of the game, children may not be able to differentiate directions rapidly. The teacher will need to gear the rapidity of the calls according to the skills of the group.

Auditory Discrimination

The following activity shows not only an active game using auditory discrimination skills, but also the way games can be adapted to other reading skills.

Concept: Auditory Discrimination — Beginning Sounds of Words

Activity: Man from Mars

One child is selected to be the man from Mars and stands in the center of the activity area. The other children stand behind a designated line at one end of the activity area. The game begins when the children call out, "Man from Mars, can we chase him through the stars?" The teacher answers, "Yes, if your name begins like duck," (or any other word). All the children whose name begins with the same beginning sound as *duck,* or whatever word is called, chase the Man from Mars until he is caught. The child who tags him becomes the new man from Mars, and the game continues.

Suggested Use: In order for the children to run at the right time, they must listen carefully and match beginning sounds. If the teacher sees a child not running when he should, individual help can be given. Children can also listen for words beginning like or ending like other words the teacher may use for the key word.

Visual Discrimination

The various games described here relating to visual discrimination indicate the variety of active game situations which can be utilized to develop skills or to assess skills development.

Concept: Visual Discrimination

Activity: Match Cats

The teacher makes duplicate sets of cards with pictures or designs on them with as many cards as there are children. The children sit on the floor. The cards are passed out randomly. On a signal or music playing, the children move around the activity area with a specified locomotor movement such as hopping or skipping. When the music stops or a signal is given, each child finds the person with his duplicate card, they join hands, with one hand and they sit on the floor together. The last couple down becomes the match cats for that turn. The children then get up and exchange cards. The game continues in the same manner using different locomotor movements.

Suggested Use: Depending on the level of skills development of the children, the cards may be pictures of real objects or abstract forms, colors, alphabet letters and words.

Concept: Visual Discrimination

Activity: Giant Step

The children stand in a line at the back of the activity area. The teacher has cards showing object pairs, similar and different. The teacher holds up one pair of cards. If the paired objects or symbols are the same, the children may take one giant step forward. Any child who moves when he sees an unpaired set of cards must return to the starting line. The object of the game is to reach the finish line opposite the activity area.

Suggested Use: The teacher may select cards to test any level of visual discrimination. Using pairs of cards for categorizing pictures would utilize concept and language development.

Concept: Visual Discrimination

Activity: Match Cards

Each child in the group is given a different-colored card. Several children are given duplicate cards. There are two chairs placed in the center of the activity area. On a signal the children may walk, skip, hop, etc., around the activity area to the music. When the music stops, the teacher holds up a card. Those children whose cards match the teacher's card run to sit in the chairs. Anyone who gets a seat scores a point, and play resumes. Cards should be exchanged frequently among the children.

Suggested Use: This visual discrimination activity can be adapted easily to include increasing complexity in the visual discrimination task how the children move and the task for scoring points. Visual discrimination tasks might also include shapes, designs and letters (both capital and lower case).

Letter Recognition

Various levels of letter recognition skills are provided for by adaptations of the following activities.

Concept: Recognizing Letter of the Alphabet

Activity: Letter Spot

Pieces of paper with lower case letters are placed in various spots around the activity area. There should be several pieces of paper with the same letters. The teacher has a number of large posters with the same but capital letters. (An overhead projector may be used to present letters in many letter styles, sizes and colors.) A poster is shown to the class. The children must identify the letter by name, then run to that letter on the floor. Any child who is left without a spot gets a point against him. Any child with less than five points at the end is considered a winner.

Suggested Use: Children are helped to associate letters with their names. After the activity the posters can be put on display around the room.

Concept: Recognizing Letters of the Alphabet
Activity: Call and Catch

The children stand in a circle. The teacher stands in the center of the circle with a rubber ball. Each child is assigned a different letter. The letter may be written on a card attached to a string which the child wears as a necklace. Each child reads his letter before the game is started. The teacher calls out a letter and throws the ball into the air. The child who has that letter tries to catch the ball after it bounces. The teacher can provide for individual differences of children. For the slower child the teacher can call the letter then momentarily hold the ball before throwing it into the air.

Suggested Use: This activity provides children the opportunity to become familiar with names and visual identification of letters. Later the teacher could hold up letter cards rather than calling the letter. The children might then have to name the letter and catch the ball. Eventually both upper and lower case cards might be used in the activity.

Diagnosis of Reading Skills

As the child moves into the beginning reading skills, motor activities continue to serve as a means both for developing and reinforcing skills as well as providing a valuable means of assessing skill mastery. Skill areas as sight vocabulary, word attack skills, alphabetical order, comprehension and vocabulary meaning can be developed through the many dimensions of motor activities described throughout this chapter. Likewise, level of skill mastery can also be assessed. Activities that utilize the various reading skills mentioned above are described in order to demonstrate the nature of activities that can be employed.

Sight Vocabulary

Developing sight vocabulary through motor activities utilizes words and phrases from materials children are currently reading.
Concept: Sight Vocabulary
Activity: Call Phrase

The children form a circle, facing the center. They may be seated or standing. One child is designated as the caller and stands in the center of the circle. Each child is given a card with a phrase printed on it. Several children can have the same phrase. The caller draws a card from a box containing corresponding phrase cards and holds up the card for everyone to see. When he reads the phrase, this is the signal for those children in the circle with the same phrase to exchange places before the caller can fill in one of the vacant places in the circle. The remaining child becomes the caller.

Suggested Use: Children need opportunities to develop quick recognition of phrases. This activity provides the repetition necessary to help children develop familiarity with phrases they are meeting in their reading material. The phrases may be taken from group experience stories, readers, or children's own experience stories.

Word Attack

Word attack skills that may be developed and assessed through motor activities may include phonic elements of words, rhyming words, vowel letter patterns, syllables and endings.

Concept: Auditory Discrimination — Consonant Digraphs (ch, sh, th)

Activity: Mouse and Cheese

A round mousetrap is formed by the children standing in a circle. In the center of the mousetrap is placed the cheese, a ball or some other object. The children are then assigned one of the consonant digraphs, *sh, ch* or *th*. When the teacher calls a word beginning with a consonant digraph, all the children with this digraph run around the circle and back to their places, representing the holes in the trap. Through these original places they run into the circle to get the cheese. The child who gets the cheese is the winning mouse for that turn. Another word is called, and the same procedure is followed. Children may be reassigned digraphs from time to time.

Suggested Use: Children need repetition for developing the ability to hear and identify various sound elements within words.

This game enables children to recognize consonant digraphs within the context of whole words. A variation of this game would be to have the teacher holdup word cards with words beginning with consonant diagraphs rather than saying the word. This variation would provide emphasis on visual discrimination of initial consonant diagraphs. Another variation would focus on ending consonant digraphs, either auditory or visual recognition.

Concept: Rhyming Words

Activity: Rhyme Chase

The children form a circle. Each child is given a card with a familiar word from the children's sight vocabulary written on it. The teacher may ask each child to pronounce his word before beginning the game. The children should listen and look at the words as each one identifies his word. The teacher then calls out a word that rhymes with one or several of the words held by the children. The child (or children) holds up his rhyming word so all the children can see it. He must then give another word that rhymes with his word. This is a signal for all the other children to run to a place of safety previously designated by the teacher. The child (or children) with the rhyming words tries to tag anyone of the other children before he reaches a safe place. A child who is tagged receives a point. The object is for the children to get the lowest scores possible. Word cards may be exchanged among the children after several turns.

Suggested Use: In this activity the children are called upon to relate auditory experiences in rhyming with visual presentations of these words. Sight vocabulary is also emphasized as the children reinforce the concept of visual patterns in rhyming words.

Alphabetical Order

Alphabetizing words is an essential skill for locating words in dictionaries or information in encyclopedias. Activities utilizing the first two, three or four letters for alphabetizing can later be developed as the teacher assesses when there is skill mastery of the less difficult tasks of alphabetizing.

Concept: Alphabetical Order

Activity: Alphabet Line-Up

The class is divided into two groups. For each group a set of twenty-six cards, one for each letter of the alphabet, is placed out of order on the chalk tray at the front of the room or pinned to a bulletin board. The groups make rows at a specified distance from the letter display. A goal line is established at the back of the room for each group. The object of the game is for each member, one at a time, to run to pick a letter in correct alphabetical order, carry it to the group's goal line, and place the letters side by side in correct order. When each group member has found a letter, the group begins again until the alphabet is complete. The first group to complete placing the alphabet correctly at its goal line wins.

Suggested Use: Children need many different types of opportunity to practice putting the letters in correct alphabetical order. This activity provides a new way to practice this skill.

Comprehension

Vocabulary meaning as well as other comprehension skills such as in the following activity utilizing a sequence of events can be emphasized in motor activities. Sentence Relay further serves as an example of how the buddy system can work in the motor activity approach.

Concept: Sequence of Events

Activity: Sentence Relay

Relay teams of five children each are selected to make rows before a starting line ten to fifteen feet from sentence charts for each team. The remaining children can serve as scorers. Each child on the team is given a sentence that fits into an overall sequence for the five sentences given a team. (The teams are given duplicate sentences.) Each sentence gives a clue to its position in the sentence sequence either by idea content or word clue. On a signal the team members get together and decide the correct sentence order. The child with the first sentence then runs to the sentence chart, places his sentence on the top line of the chart, underlines the key part of the sentence that gives the clue to the sequence, and returns to his team. The child with the next sentence then runs to place his sentence below the first sentence. This procedure continues until the sentences are in order. The team to complete the story with the sentences in correct order first wins. The scorers check on the accuracy of the sentence order for each team. For the next game the scorers can exchange places with those who were on teams. Variations of this activity can include the use of cartoons with each child being given one frame of the cartoon strip. To make the activity more difficult, more sentences may be added to the sequence. To prevent copying, the teacher can give different story sentences to each team.

Suggested Use: In this activity those children having difficulty with reading are helped by those who are more able readers and not eliminated from the game. After each game the teacher should go over key elements in the sentences that provided clues to the proper sequence.

How might Sentence Relay be used for diagnostic purposes? It might be used just as it is described above or certain adaptations might be made. In this case, the reading task in the activity is to recognize key elements in the sentences that provide clues to the proper sequence. The teacher can notice whether a child is able to identify appropriate clues to sequence in his sentence. The teacher might observe which children perform the task easily and those who appear to need additional experiences in identifying key elements in sentences relating to sequence.

The activity might also be adapted by changing the game to one that utilizes a story with several key sentences missing, the number of missing sentences being the same as the number of children on each team. The reading would then be one of using context clues of a large meaning unit to identify the proper order of sentences.

One of the many advantages of the motor activity approach is that it is fairly easy for the teacher to identify the specific reading skills being utilized in a game which in turn facilitates assessment of children's mastery of that skill. In this way diagnostic teaching techniques aid a teacher's efforts to adjust the learning activities of the reading program to the needs of the children. The examples presented here are representative of almost unlimited possibilities in structuring appropriate reading experiences for children. The creative teacher should be able to develop numerous activities by adapting those presented in the present text to the developmental level and skill needs of the children.

SELECTED MOTOR ACTIVITIES TO
TEACH READING SKILLS

The following is a summary of motor activities that contain reading and language arts concepts and skills. They include a variety of representative examples of the numerous possibilities. Teachers are encouraged to use their own ingenuity in adding to this list. Descriptions of the activities follow the summary.

Concept	*Activity*
Word Analysis Skills:	
Recognizing Letters of the Alphabet	Letter Snatch
Auditory Discrimination	Match The Sound
Consonant Blends, Consonant Digraphs,	Crows and Cranes
Vowels	Call Blends
	Final Blend Change
Initial Consonant Substitution	First Letter Change
Visual Discrimination	See The Same
Whole Words	Cross The Bridge
Auditory and Visual Association	Consonant Relay
Initial Consonants	
Inflectional Endings	Ending Relay
Accent	Accent Relay
Alphabetical Order	Alphabet Relay
Comprehension:	
Following Directions	Simon Says
	Do This, Do That
Vocabulary Meaning	Match The Meaning
	Rainbow
	The Mulberry Bush
	Over and Under Relay
	What To Play
	Action Relay
	Word Change
	I'm Tall, I'm Small

Word Analysis Skills

Concept: Recognizing Letters of the Alphabet
Activity: Letter Snatch

The children are divided into two teams of ten each. The teams face each other about ten to twelve feet apart. A small object such as an eraser is placed on the floor between the two teams. The members of both teams are given like letters. The teacher then holds up a card with a letter on it. The children from each team who have the letter run out and try to grab the object and return to their line. If the child does so without being tagged by the other child, he scores two points. If he is tagged, the other team scores one point.

Suggested Use: Children have the opportunity to practice letter recognition in this activity. Visual matching can be with all small letters at first, then later with all capital letters. After the children have learned both small and capital letters, one team can have small letters and the other, capital letters, with the teacher displaying cards showing either type of letter.

Concept: Auditory Discrimination — Beginning Sounds in Words

Activity: Match The Sound

A group of eight to ten children form a circle. The children skip around in the circle until the teacher gives a signal to stop. The teacher then says a word and throws a ball to one of the children. The teacher begins to count to ten. The child who catches the ball must say another word which begins with the same sound before the teacher counts to ten. If the child does, he gets a point. The child with the most points wins. The other children in the circle must listen carefully to be sure each child calls out a correct word. As the children learn to associate letter names with sounds, the child must not only call another word beginning with the same sound, but must identify the letter that word begins with.

Suggested Use: This activity enables children to listen for sounds in the initial position of words. The game can also be adapted to listening for final position sounds.

Concept: Auditory Discrimination — Consonant Blends

Activity: Crows and Cranes

The activity area is divided by a center line. On opposite ends of the area are drawn base lines parallel to the center line. The class is divided into two teams. The children of one team are designated as crows and take position on one side of the activity area, with the base line on their side of the center line serving as their safety zone. The members of the other team are designated as cranes and take position on the other side of the activity area with their base line as a safety zone. The teacher stands to one side of the activity area by the center line. The teacher then calls out, Cr-r-anes or Cr-rows. In calling cranes or crows, the teacher emphasizes the initial consonant blend. If the teacher calls the crows, they turn and run to their base line to avoid being tagged by the cranes. The cranes attempt to tag their opponents before they can cross their base line. The cranes score a point for each crow tagged. The crows and cranes then return to their places, and the teacher proceeds to call one of the groups; play continues in the same manner. This game can be extended to include other words beginning with consonant blends, for example, swans and swallows, storks and starlings, squids and squabs.

Suggested Use: Repetition of the consonant blends during the game helps children become aware of these sounds and to develop their auditory perception of the blends in the context of words. Discovering names of animals with other consonant blends can help children in their ability to hear consonant blends in the initial position of words.

Concept: Auditory Discrimination — Consonant Blends
Activity: Call Blends

Eight to ten children stand in a circle. The teacher stands in the center of the circle, holding a ball. Each child is assigned an initial consonant blend by the teacher (st, gr, bl, cl and so forth). When the teacher calls out a word with an initial consonant blend, the ball is thrown into the air. The child assigned that blend must then call a word using the blend and catch the ball after it has bounced once. Depending on the ability level of the children, the teacher can control the amount of time between calling out the blend word and the time the child catches the ball and calls out his word. Then the child gives a correct word and catches the ball, he scores one point. The child with the most points wins. The teacher can reassign blends frequently to the children during the game.

Suggested Use: This activity is a supplemental one to reinforce previous auditory and visual presentation of consonant blends in the initial position. Blends used should be those with which the children have worked. The teacher may write the word on the board after each time and have the child underline the blend in order to reinforce the blend in the visual context of the word.

Concept: Auditory Discrimination — Final Consonant Blends

(nk, ck, nd, st, nt, rst)

Activity: Final Blend Change

The children form a single circle with one child standing in the center of the circle. The children in the circle are designated as different final consonant blends. Several children will be assigned the same blends. Each child may be given a card with his blend written on it to help him remember. The teacher then pronounces a word with one of the final position blends. All the children with this blend must hold up their card, then run to exchange places. The child in the center tries to get one of the vacant places in the circle. The remaining child goes to the center.

Suggested Use: This activity helps children to develop their auditory discrimination of final position blends. They must listen carefully to the words pronounced. By holding up their cards, they are associating the visual with the auditory symbol for that sound. The teacher may write the word down that is called out and have one of the children underline the final consonant blend so they can see the blend in the context of the whole word.

Concept: Initial Consonant Substitution

Activity: First Letter Change

The class is divided into several teams. The teams stand in rows behind a starting line some ten to fifteen feet from the chalkboard. A word such as *ball* is written on the board for each team. (To prevent copying, different words should be used for each team.) On a signal the first child on each team goes to the board; says the word; writes another word, changing the intial consonant to make another meaningful word; says the word; then runs to the rear of his team. The second child of the team repeats this same sequence. The first team to complete the writing of words with initial consonant substitution correctly scores a point. Any child having trouble may ask the help of one member of his team to identify another word.

Suggested Use: Children are able to develop their skills in using initial consonant substitution in this activity with the added dimension of visual and kinesthetic experiences by seeing a word and writing new words, using different intial consonants.

Concept: Visual Discrimination — Whole Words

Activity: See the Same

The children are divided into two groups. Sets of word cards are made up and placed in a large, shallow box, one for each team. The words selected are those being developed as sight vocabulary. A pair of word cards is made up for each word. The words are then mixed up in the boxes. The two teams stand in rows behind a starting line. On a signal the first child of each group runs to the group's box and looks for two words that are alike. He then displays the pair of words on a sentence chart holder that is set up next to the group's box. The next child in the group proceeds in the same manner. The first group which has each child find a pair of words wins. A child having difficulty may seek the help from one member of his group.

Suggested Use: Children need opportunities to visually match not only letters, but also words in order for them to develop the skills of seeing letter elements within the gestalt of the whole word. This activity provides an interesting means for developing this skill. The teacher may encourage the children to identify the word pair they have found. (If there are additional sentence chart holders, it is desirable to have smaller groups and, thus, more teams.)

Concept: Visual Discrimination — Whole Words
Activity: Cross the Bridge

The activity area is marked off with lines at each end. A child is selected to be the bridge keeper. He stands in the center of the area while the remainder of the class stands behind one end line. Each child is given a card with a sight vocabulary word on it. Several children should have the same word. The bridge keeper is given a box with a complete set of word cards that correspond to those given the other children. They must be large enough for all the children to see. The children call out to the bridge keeper, "May we use the bridge?" The bridge keeper replies, "Yes, if you are this word." He then holds up one of the word cards from his box for all the children to see. The child or children having that word try to cross to the other end line without being tagged by the bridge keeper. The procedure is continued again with other words. Those children tagged must help the bridge keeper tag the other children as they also try to cross the bridge. Occasionally, the bridge keeper may call out, "Everybody cross the bridge," when all the children may then run to the opposite end line. The game can continue until one child remains. He becomes the bridge keeper for the next game, or another bridge keeper may be selected.

Suggested Use: This activity provides children the opportunity to match words visually as a means to reinforce words to the point that they may become a part of the child's sight vocabulary.

Concept: Auditory and Visual Association — Initial Consonants
Activity: Consonant Relay

The children are divided into several relay teams. The teams line up at a specified distance from a chalkboard and are seated. The teacher stands so as to be seen by the children when pronouncing the words. The teacher says a word beginning with a consonant sound. The last child in each team runs to the board, writes the beginning consonant and returns to the head of his team. Each child moves back one place. The first child to get back to his seat with the correct letter written on the board scores a point for his team. The teacher says another word, and the game continues as above until everyone has had a turn. The team with the highest score wins.

Suggested Use: This activity gives children practice in hearing initial consonant sounds and associating them with their written symbols. This game can be adapted to working with final consonants, digraphs, blends and long and short vowels.

Concept: Inflectional Endings — *s, ed, ing*
Activity: Ending Relay

The class is divided into teams. Each team is given a box filled with sight vocabulary words having *s, ed* and *ing* endings. The boxes are placed by a chalkboard. The teams make rows at a starting line ten to fifteen feet from the chalkboard. On a signal the first child of each team runs to the team's box and picks out three words, one with an *s* ending, one with an *ed* ending, and one with an *ing* ending. He places the words along the chalk tray, pronounces each and returns to his team. The second child continues in the same manner. If a child is having difficulty, he may call upon one member of his team to help him. The team that finishes with the accurate selection and pronunciation of words first wins.

Suggested Use: This activity enables children to practice their skills in identifying visually presented words with different inflectional endings. This activity also provides reinforcement of sight vocabulary.

Concept: Accent as Cues to Meaning

Activity: Accent Relay

The class is divided into several teams. The teams make rows behind a starting line ten to fifteen feet from a chalkboard. Complete sets of words (a few more than the number of children on the teams), divided into syllables and marked with accents, are written on the board. Examples of words to be used are *ob'ject* and *object' re'cord* and *record'*, and *per'mit* and *permit'*. The teacher reads a sentence in which one of the words from the board is used. The first child on each team runs to the board and underlines the correct word as it was used in the teacher's sentence. He then returns to the rear of his team. The first child to return to his team scores a point for his team. The second child proceeds to underline a second word with the teacher's reading of another sentence. This procedure continues until each child has an opportunity to participate. The team with the most points wins. At any time a child is having difficulty, he may ask one member of his team for help.

Suggested Use: This activity helps children to listen carefully to words in the context of a sentence for clues to meaning. Children can also be helped to notice the change of the function of these words in sentences when there is an accent change, that of moving from a noun to a verb function.

Concept: Alphabetical Order

Activity: Alphabet Relay

The children are divided into several teams. Word lists are written on the board for each team with as many words as there are team members. There should be different words in each list. The teams make rows behind a starting line ten to fifteen from the chalkboard. On a signal the first child on each team runs to the board and writes the number 1 in front of the first word in alphabetical order. Upon returning to the rear of his team, the second child runs and puts number 2 in front of the second word to come in alphabetical order. This procedure is continued until all the words are numbered in proper alphabetical order. The first team completing its list correctly wins. The difficulty of the alphabetizing task can be increased by using words with the same first letter, then the same first two letters and so on. A child who is having difficulty may seek the help from one member of his team. *Suggested Use:* This highly motivating activity provides children with the necessary repetition for developing skills of alphabetizing words. The nature of the competition also puts emphasis on quickness in using this skill as an aid to finding words in a dictionary in a minimum amount of time.

Comprehension

Concept: Following Directions
Activity: Simon Says

The children stand about the activity area facing the person who plays Simon. Every time Simon says to do something, the children must do it. However, if a command is given without the prefix "Simon says," the children must remain motionless. For example, when "Simon says take two jumps," everyone must take two jumps, but if Simon says, "Walk backward two steps," no one should move. If a child moves at the wrong time or turns in the wrong direction, the child puts one hand on his head. The second time he misses he puts the other hand on his head. The next time he misses, an additional forfeit is assigned. The more quickly the commands are given and the greater number of commands, the more difficult the game will be. The child with the least number of misses is the winner.
Suggested Use: This activity provides children the opportunity to follow oral directions in a highly motivating situation. The rules of the game as adapted allow those children who need practice additional chances to remain in the game rather than be eliminated. It might be desirable to divide the class into teams, with the team having the least number of misses after a specified period of time be the winner.
Concept: Following Directions
Activity: Do This, Do That

Flash cards of "Do This" and "Do That" are used in this activity. One child is selected to be the leader and stands in front of the group. The teacher holds up a flash card, and the leader makes a movement such as walking in place, running in place, swinging his arms or hopping. The children follow the actions of the leader when the sign says "Do This." When the teacher holds up the sign "Do That," the children must not move, although the leader continues the action. A point is scored against the child who is caught moving. The object of the game is to get the lowest score possible. The leader can be changed frequently.

Suggested Use: This activity can be used to help children to read carefully in order to follow directions. Later, this activity can be adapted by having the leader display written directions on flash cards, for example hop in place, jump once, run in place and the like.

Concept: Vocabulary Meaning

Activity: Match The Meaning

The children are divided into several teams. The teams make rows ten to fifteen feet from the chalkboard. Meanings of words are written on the board ahead of time, a group of definitions for each team. Each child is given a card with a word that matches a meaning on the board. On a signal the first child runs to the board and erases the meaning that defines the word. The child may seek the help of his team before going to the board. The teacher checks each child before he erases his definition. If the child still has selected a definition that is incorrect, he must return to his team so they can decide what the correct definition is. Each child proceeds in the same manner until every child has identified the definition of his word and has returned to his team. The first team to finish wins.

Suggested Use: Emphasis needs to be placed on word meanings when developing sight vocabulary. This activity provides an exciting and highly motivating means of providing practice with meanings, and children are able to help each other develop word meanings. The activity may be set up for specific reading groups to reinforce words they are meeting in their stories.

Concept: Vocabulary Meaning — Colors

Activity: Rainbow

The children form a circle facing the center. They may be seated or standing. One child is designated the caller and stands in the center of the circle. Instead of counting off by numbers, the children are given a small piece of paper of one of the basic colors. The caller is given a set of word cards, one for each of the basic colors corresponding to the colors given the children in the circle. The caller selects one word card and shows it. The children with this color attempt to change places while the caller tries to get one of the vacant places in the circle. The remaining child becomes the new caller. The caller may show two word cards. Those children with the two colors then run to change places with the caller again, trying to get to one of the vacant places in the circle. At any time the caller or teacher may call out, Rainbow! When this call is given, everyone must change to a different position. *Suggested Use:* Children need many opportunities to develop their recognition of words in activities of this nature in which they are associating the word and the concept the word represents. This game can be simplified in order for it to become appropriate for a language development activity. The caller can have just color cards matching those of the children. Later, when the children have learned to match colors, the caller can call out the names of the colors.

Concept: Vocabulary Meanings — Action Words and Days of the Week

Activity: Mulberry Bush

   The children form a circle, facing in. The teacher may write the days of the week on the board in proper order and go over them with the children before the activity is begun. The teacher can also talk with the children about how they would do the various tasks involved in the various verses. As the verses are sung, the children act out the action of the words.

> Here we go round the mulberry bush,
> The mulberry bush, the mulberry bush,
> Here we go round the mulberry bush,
> So early in the morning.
> This is the way we wash our clothes,
> Wash our clothes, wash our clothes,
> This is the way we wash our clothes,
> So early Monday morning.
> This is the way we iron our clothes,

etc.

So early Tuesday morning.

This is the way we mend our clothes,

etc.

So early Wednesday morning.

This is the way we scrub the floor,

etc.

So early Thursday morning.

This is the way we sweep the house,

etc.

So early Friday morning.

This is the way we bake our bread,

etc.

So early Saturday morning.

This is the way we go to church,

etc.

So early Sunday morning.

Suggested Use: This activity helps children recall the days of the week in their proper order. It also helps children to develop the concept that words represent action or behavior of people that can be observed, as well as names of specific objects.

Concept: Vocabulary Meaning — Over and Under

Activity: Over and Under Relay

The children are divided into several teams. The children stand one behind the other, separated about one foot apart. A ball is given to the first child of each team. On a signal the first child passes the ball behind him over his head and calls, "Over." The second child takes the ball and passes it between his legs and calls, "Under." This continues until the last child receives the ball. He then runs to the head of his column and starts passing the ball back in the same manner. The team whose first child reaches the head of the column first wins.

Suggested Use: This activity helps children to dramatize the meaning of the words *over* and *under*. For a variation the teacher can hold up a card with either *over* or *under* written on it to indicate how the first child on each team should start passing the ball or how the ball should be passed by the child moving forward to the front of the team.

Concept: Vocabulary Meaning — Action Words
Activity: What To Play

The children stand near their desks. One of the children is selected to be the leader. While that child is coming to the front of the room to lead, the rest of the class begins to sing, to the tune of "Mary Had a Little Lamb,"

> Mary tell us what to play,
> What to play, what to play,
> Mary tell us what to play,
> Tell us what to play.

The leader then says, "Let's play we're fishes," (or any kind of activity). The leader then performs the action that the other children imitate. On a signal the children stop, and a new leader is selected.

Suggested Use: This activity gives children an opportunity to act out the meanings of words. It helps them to recognize that spoken words represent actions of people as well as things that can be touched.

Concept: Vocabulary Meaning — Action Words
Activity: Action Relay

The children divide into several teams. The teams make rows ten to fifteen feet from the chalkboard. The teacher makes duplicate lists for each team with as many action words on the board for each team as there are team members. The first child on each team, on a signal, runs to the board, crosses out the first word, calls it out, and does what the word says as he returns to his team and touches the next child. The second child proceeds in the same manner until every child has demonstrated a word. Any child who cannot figure out his word can ask one member of his team to help him. The first team to complete the acting out of each word correctly, wins.

Suggested Use: This activity helps children to build meanings of words by having them dramatize the words. This helps children to visualize the meanings of words. Children who are having difficulty should not be eliminated from the game, but should receive help from the other children.

Concept: Vocabulary Meaning — Word Opposites
Activity: Word Change

The class is divided into two teams who line up at opposite ends of the activity area. Each child is given a word printed on a card. The words given to one team are the word opposites of the words given to the other team. One child is selected to be *it* and stands in the middle of the activity area. The teacher calls out a word, and this word and its opposite run and try to exchange places. *It* attempts to get into one of the vacated places before the two children can exchange places. The remaining child becomes *it* for the next time.

Suggested Use: This activity focuses on the meaning of sight vocabulary words. It can be varied with emphasis on synonyms, with the teams given words that are similar in meaning.

Concept: Vocabulary Meaning — Word Opposites

Activity: I'm Tall, I'm Small

The children form a circle with one child in the center. The child in the center of the circle stands with his eyes closed. It may be helpful to have the child blindfolded. The children in the circle walk around the circle singing or saying the following verse:

> I'm tall, I'm very small,
> I'm small, I'm very tall,
> Sometimes I'm tall,
> Sometimes I'm small,
> Guess what I am now.

As the children walk and sing, tall, very tall, or small or very small, they stretch up or stoop down, depending on the words. At the end of the singing the teacher signals the children in the circle to assume a stretching or stooping position. The child in the center, still with eyes closed, guesses which position they have taken. For the next time another child is selected to be in the center.

Suggested Use: This activity helps children to develop word meaning by acting out the words. Use of word opposites in this manner helps to dramatize the differences in the meaning of words. The words and actions can be changed to incorporate a larger number of opposites, for example

> My hands are near, my hands are far,
> Now they're far, now they're near,
> Sometimes they're near,

Sometimes they're far,
Guess what they are now.

It should be repeated again that the activities presented here are representative examples of an infinite number of possibilities. Teachers should consider variations of these learning activities for specific situations as well as to devise activities of their own.

CHAPTER SIX

LEARNING ABOUT MATHEMATICS THROUGH MOTOR ACTIVITY

WHEN the so-called *new math* was introduced into the American educational system in the early 1960's, it was probably one of the greatest upheavals in curriculum content and procedures in modern times. In any event it has been heralded as such. In general, the *new math* was intended to do away with a process that had focused upon rote memory and meaningless computation. Further, it was expected that the new process would facilitate for students the development of mathematical understandings.

The extent to which the *new math* has achieved success has been challenged by educators and laymen alike. Obviously, most educational innovations have rightly been criticized when one gives consideration to the extremes that are possible in any educational process. Because of this, it now appears that attempts are being made to reach some sort of happy medium. This is to say that it is not likely that anyone wishes to revert entirely to the *old math*, at the same time, it would be desirable to avoid some of the extremes that have brought harsh criticism of the *new math*.

In some instances, efforts are being made to "avoid the hazards of meaningless memory work and number manipulations on the one hand and dry theory on the other."[1] It is said that an approach such as this would be more suited to the everyday facts of life.

It is the belief of the present author that the motor activity approach to learning about mathematics not only deals with the everyday facts of life, *but with life itself.* This chapter is devoted to ways and means by which this may be accomplished.

_____
[1] World Progress Report, Number games. *Saturday Review World*, September 7, 1974.

SOME GENERAL WAYS OF PROVIDING MATHEMATICS
EXPERIENCES THROUGH MOTOR ACTIVITY

There are numerous motor learning activities for use of such processes as counting, computing and measuring inherent in various types of motor activities. Although it is the primary purpose of this chapter to deal essentially with more or less *specific* ways to learn about mathematics through motor activity, mention is made here about how this can occur *generally* in such broad categories of motor activities as *game* activities, *rhythmic* activities and *self-testing* activities.

Mathematics Learning Experiences in Game Activities

In certain types of games, such as tag games where a certain number of children are caught, the number of children caught can be counted. After determining the number caught, pupils can be asked how many were left. The number caught can be added to the number left to check for the correct answer. In this procedure counting, adding and subtracting are utilized as number experiences in the game activity. An example of this is shown in the game Lions and Tigers.

In this game the class is divided into two equal groups. One group is the lions and the other, the tigers. Each group stands on a goal line at opposite ends of the activity area. Both groups face in the same direction. To start the game the lions come up behind the tigers as quietly as possible. The tigers listen for the lions, and when it is determined from the sound that they are near, one person who has been designated calls out, the lions are coming. The tigers turn, give chase and try to tag as many as they can before the lions reach their own goal line. Those caught can become members of the opposite group. The above procedure is reversed and the game proceeds.

In one situation this game was used for a better understanding of *comparison of groups and more or less*. The class was working on the one-to-one relationship between groups. This game gave the class another opportunity to use this concept in a real situation. The children understood that each team would try to add to their players. The winner was determined by counting the lions and tigers. There were eighteen lions and twelve tigers. The lions and tigers stood in a line, face to face, to get another demonstration of the one-to-one concept. There were some lions who did not have a tiger to face as the lion line was longer. The class was able to see clearly that one group was larger than the other. This group had *more* children in it; the other had *less*. The lion line was longer than the tiger line. The class drew the following conclusions: The higher we count, the bigger the number. Therefore, 18 is more than 12; 12 is less than 18; 9 is more than 6; and 6 is less than 9. The class made many such group comparisons.

In those types of games that require scoring, for example, the number of runs scored in a baseball-type game, there are opportunities for counting, adding and subtracting as well as the use of fractions. Pupils can compute how many *more* runs one group scored and how many *fewer* runs another group scored. Teachers may find it useful to count a score with a number in which the class needs practice in adding. For example, a score could count five points and the number five would be added whenever a score was made. Also, use may be made of one base being one fourth of the way around the bases; two bases one half of a run and so on to demonstrate in a concrete way the use of fractions.

In games in which children have a number and go into action when their numbers are called, mathematics can be used by having the leader who calls the number give a problem which will have as its answer the number of the players who are to go into action. Any of the four processes of addition, subtraction, multiplication or division, or any combination of these may be used.

An example of such a game is Club Snatch. It is played with two teams of from eight to sixteen players on a team, forming two lines facing each other about ten to twelve feet apart. An object such as a ten pin or a beanbag is placed in the middle of the space between the two lines. The team members are numbered from opposite directions. The teacher or a pupil acting as the leader calls a number, and each of the two players with that number runs out and tries to grab the object and return to his line. If the player does so, his team scores two points; if he is tagged by his opponent, the other team scores one point. The teacher might give a problem in the following manner, "Ready! 10 minus 2, divided by 4, times 3, plus 1, Go!" The answer would be 7; the two players having this number would attempt to retrieve the object. Care should be taken to have competing children as nearly equal as possible.

Mathematics Learning Experiences in Rhythmic Activities

There are many rhythmic activities in which mathematics experiences are inherent. A case in point is the singing game, Ten Little Indians. In this activity the children form a circle, all facing in. Ten children are selected to be Indians, and numbered from one to ten. As the song is sung, the child whose number is called skips to the center of the circle. When ten little Indians are in the center, the song is reversed. Again, each child leaves the center and returns to the circle as his number is called. Other children may become Indians, and the song is repeated. The words to the song are

> One little, two little, three little Indians,
> Four little, five little, six little Indians,
> Seven little, eight little, nine little Indians,
> Ten little Indian boys (or girls).
> Ten little, nine little, eight little Indians,
> Seven little, six little, five little Indians,
> Four little, three little, two little Indians,
> One little Indian boy.

This activity can be used to develop the understanding of *quantitative aspects of numbers and counting*. Position and sequence of numbers is important in basic mathematics concepts. In this rhythmic activity children can be helped to see the quantitative aspects of ordinal numbers, and the subtraction concept may also be introduced through this activity.

In a few instances materials have been especially prepared in the form of rhythmic activities to develop certain mathematics concepts. A case in point is the following example of some of the work by the present author.[2]

The name of this rhythmic activity is Take Away, Take Away. The children stand in a circle and one child is *it*. This child walks around inside the circle. As the children sing the following song, to the tune of "Twinkle Twinkle Little Star," they act out the words of the song.

> Take away, take away, take away one.
> Come with me and have some fun.
> Take away, take away, take away two.
> Come with me, oh yes please do.
> Take away, take away, take away three.
> All please come and skip with me.

It taps one child. This child follows behind *it*. *It* then taps a second and third child. At the end of the song all three children try to get back to their places in the circle. *It* also tries to get into one of the vacant places. The remaining child becomes *it* if the activity is continued. This activity has been used very successfully because it enables children to see demonstrated the concept of subtraction. The teacher may have the children identify how many are left each time *it* takes away one child.

Mathematics Learning Experiences in Self-Testing Activities

Numbers can satisfactorily be incorporated in a variety of ways in the teaching of certain self-testing activities and motor skills. For example, counting can be facilitated for young children when it is done by counting the number of times they bounced a ball. Addition and subtraction can be brought in here also by having them compute the number of times they bounced the ball one time and how many more or fewer times they bounced it another time. This same procedure can be applied to activities such as rope jumping as indicated by the following examples:

Let the rope swing forward seven times before you jump over it. Joan, after the rope turns five times, you run in and jump nine times.

Because so many stunt activities can be broken down into a

---

[2]James H. Humphrey, *Teaching Children Mathematics Through Games, Rhythms, and Stunts.* LP 5000, Deal, Kimbo Educational, 1968.

number of parts, there is an opportunity to teach about fractions in connection with these kinds of activities. An example is the Squat Thrust which is performed in the following manner. From a standing position the child assumes a squatting stance, placing the hands on the surface area to the outside of the legs with the palms flat and the fingers pointed forward. This is the first count. On the second count the weight is shifted to the hands and arms, and the legs are extended sharply to the rear until the body is straight. The weight of the body is now on the hands and the balls of the feet. On the third count the child returns to the squatting position, and on the fourth count the child returns to the erect standing position.

In teaching this stunt with reference to fractional parts of a whole (1/4, 1/2, 3/4) as well as addition of fractions, the following auditory input might be furnished in connection with the performance of the stunt.

> Here is a stunt with four parts. First you stand straight with feet together. Hands are at your side. Next you stoop down to a squat position. Your hands are in front on the floor. Now you have done the first part of the stunt. You have done one fourth of the stunt. Next you kick way back with your feet. Now you have done one half of the stunt. Next you bring your legs back to the squat position. Now you have done three fourths of the stunt. Next you stand up straight again. Now you have done the whole stunt.

As additional input the teacher can make a circle out of cardboard and cut it into one fourths. As the child does each part of the stunt the one fourths can be put together. Another variation would be to draw a circle on the floor. The child makes his movements in the circle, calling out the fractional parts as he does so.

THE MATHEMATICS MOTOR ACTIVITY STORY

Widespread success resulting from the use of motor-oriented reading content discussed in the previous chapter inspired the development of the same general type of reading content which would also include mathematics experiences. This kind of reading content was arbitrarily called *the mathematics motor activity story.*

Early attempts to develop mathematics motor activity stories were patterned after the original procedure used in providing for motor-oriented reading content — that is several stories were written around certain kinds of motor activities, the only difference being that the content also involved reference to mathematics experiences. These stories were tried out in a number of situations. It soon became apparent that with some children the understanding of the mathematics concept(s) in a story was too difficult. The reason for this appeared to be that certain children could not handle both the task of reading while at the same time developing an understanding of the mathematics aspect of the story. It was then decided that since *listening* is a first step in learning to read, auditory input should be utilized. This procedure involved having children listen to a story, perform the activity and simultaneously try to develop the mathematics concept. When it appeared desirable, this process was extended by having the children read the story after having engaged in the activity. Following is a description of one of our first experiences with a mathematics motor activity story.[3]

The following story was written by the author and used and evaluated by a first grade teacher with her class of thirty children. The name of the story is Find a Friend and it is an adaptation of a game called BUSY BEE. The readability level of the story is 1.5 (fifth month of first grade). The mathematics concepts inherent in the story are: *Groups or sets of two; counting by twos; beginning concept of multiplication.*

Find A Friend

> In this game each child finds a friend.
> Stand beside your friend.
> You and your friend make a group of two.
> One child is *it*.
> He does not stand beside a friend.
> He calls, Move!

---

[3]James H. Humphrey, The mathematics motor activity story. *The Arithmetic Teacher*, January, 1967.

All friends find a new friend.
It tries to find a friend.
The child who does not find a friend is *it*.
Play the game.
Count the number of friends standing together.
Count by two.
Say two, four, six.
Count all the groups this way.

The group of first grade children with whom this experiment was conducted bordered on the remedial level and had no previous experience in counting by twos. Before the activity, each child was checked for the ability to count by twos; it was found that none had it. Also, the children had no previous classroom experience with beginning concepts of multiplication.

The story was read to the children and the directions were discussed. The game was demonstrated by the teacher and several children. Five pairs of children were used at one time. As the game was being played, the activity was stopped momentarily, and the child who was *it* at that moment was asked to count the groups by twos. The participants were then changed, the number participating changed, and the activity was repeated.

In evaluating the experiment it was found that this was a very successful experience from a learning standpoint. Before the activity none of the children were able to count by twos. A check following the activity showed that eighteen of the thirty children who participated in the game were able to count rationally to ten by twos. Seven children were able to count rationally to six, and two were able to count to four. Three children showed no understanding of the concept. No attempt was made to check beyond ten because in playing the game the players were limited to numbers under ten.

There appeared to be a significant number of children who had profited from this experience in a very short period of time. The teacher maintained that, in a more conventional teaching situation, the introduction and development of this concept with children at this low a level of ability would have taken a great deal more teaching time, and the results would have been attained at a much slower rate.

Several experiments similar to the one presented above were conducted with much the same results. With such information at hand it was decided to attempt a more objective approach in order to compare the use of the mathematics motor activity story with more traditional ways of teaching mathematics. To this end some objective studies were conducted, one of which is reported here.[4]

Two groups of second grade children with twenty-one in one group and twenty-three in the other group were pretested on two-number addition facts, three-number addition equations, and subtraction facts. The test contained forty-five items.

One group of children, designated as the experimental group, was taught through six mathematics motor activities stories of the type illustrated previously. The other group, designated as the control group, was taught through such traditional procedures as the printed number line, plastic discs and abstract algorisms. The experiment was conducted over a four-day period, and both groups were taught by the same classroom teacher. Each group was characterized by heterogeneity as far as age and IQ were concerned.

At the end of the four-day period both groups, having been taught the processes as indicated above, were retested. Comparisons of the pre and posttest scores were evaluated, and at an extended interval of ten days after the posttest, the test was given again with the same statistical procedures applied to the posttest and extended interval test. The range of scores on the pretest for the experimental group was 12 to 44 with a mean of 30.48, and for the control group, 4 to 44 with a mean of 30.87. The posttest scores of the experimental group ranged from 18 to 45 with a mean of 37.77, while the posttest scores of the control group ranged from 5 to 44 with a mean of 34.91. In the experimental group the range of scores on the extended interval test was from 7 to 45 with a mean of 40.50, and in the control group, from 15 to 45 with a mean of 39.7. The gain from pretest to posttest favored the experimental group at a high level of probability. Essentially the same results were obtained in gain

---

[4]James H. Humphrey, Comparison of the use of the physical education learning medium with traditional procedures in the development of certain arithmetical processes with second-grade children. *Research Abstracts*, A.A.H.P.E.R., Washington, D. C., 1968.

from posttest to extended interval test.

In recognition of various limitations imposed by a study of this nature, any conclusions should be characterized by caution. If one accepts the levels of significant differences in the test scores as evidence of learning, these second grade children could develop certain number processes better and perhaps retain them longer through use of the mathematics motor activity story rather than through some of the traditional procedures.

Finally, it seems pertinent to mention certain observations which would not show up in a statistical analysis. It was noticed that the children in the experimental group appeared to be stimulated by the use of the mathematics motor activity story. In fact, some of them commented, We didn't have arithmetic today. This could possibly mean that the learning activities were enjoyed to the extent that the children might not have been aware of the particular number skills they were using. It is worthy of comment also that several of the children in the experimental group seemed to have little or no interest in any of their arithmetic work until after they got into the experiences provided by the mathematics motor activity stories.

After considerable experimentation with the mathematics motor activity stories as indicated in the preceding discussion, materials were produced for widespread use as follows:

James H. Humphrey: *Teaching Children Mathematics Through Games, Rhythms, and Stunts.* LP No. 5000, Deal, Kimbo Educational, 1968.

This material consists of two long-play records of mathematics motor activity stories and a teacher's manual which provides suggestions for use of the material. The manual provides for general ways to use the material and more detailed specific ways for each individual selection. When a teacher plans to use a given selection, all of the information connected with it should be read very carefully. This information consists of (1) a story written at a specific reading level, (2) the mathematical skills, concepts and learnings inherent in the story, and (3) suggested ways of developing the skills, concepts and learnings with children. Following is a representative example of the material.

This example involves the game of Mouse Trap, and the story

written about this game has a reading level of 1.7. (The first number refers to grade, and the second number refers to months. Thus, 1.7 means seventh month of first grade.)

Mrs. Brown's Mouse Trap

Some of the children stand in a ring.
They hold hands.
They hold them high.
This will be a mouse trap.
The other children are mice.
They go in and out of the ring.
One child will be Mrs. Brown.
She will say, Snap!
Children drop hands.
The mouse trap closes.
Some mice will be caught.
Count them.
Tell how many.
Tell how many were not caught.
Play again.

Mathematical Skills and Concepts

Rational counting
Addition
Subtraction

Teaching Suggestions

1. All of the children can count together the number caught.
2. All of the children can count together the number not caught.
3. If the teacher wishes, he or she can have the children who are caught stand in a line facing those not caught. This way the children can easily see the difference.

SELECTED MOTOR ACTIVITIES FOR DEVELOPING MATHEMATICS CONCEPTS

The motor activities in the ensuing section of the chapter have been grouped by some of the major areas of the elementary school mathematics curriculum. The summation of each activity indicates the inherent mathematics concept or number skills involved. Some of the activities are particularly useful for introducing and developing a mathematics concept. These involve the learner actively, and provide the child the opportunity to act out the concept physically. Other activities reinforce a concept and develop skills by providing the practice children might need, but in an interesting and personally involving situation.

In the "Suggested Use" section for each activity the teacher is provided suggestions for using the activity to develop the concept inherent in the activity. If the activity is more appropriate for reinforcement of a concept previously developed, the section on suggested use specifies the skills being developed through practice and use in a highly motivating situation. The teacher will no doubt want to adapt many of the activities to develop mathematics concepts or practice arithmetic skills other than the ones utilized in the activities as presented.

Classification of Motor Activities According to Major Areas in Elementary School Mathematics

The following is a summary of motor activities that contain mathematics concepts and skills. Descriptions of the activities follow the summary.

Concept	*Activity*
Number System:	
Quantitative Aspects of Numbers and Numeral Recognition	Watch the Numbers
Quantitative Aspects of Numbers and Counting	Bee Sting
	Count and Go
	Muffin Man
	Fish Net
	Round Up
	Chain Tag
	Come With Me
	Ball Pass
Counting	Count, Move and Stop
	Pick-Up Race

	Pass Ball Relay
	Red Light
Ordinal Numbers	Leader Ball
	The Number Race
Addition:	Three Deep
	Back to Back
	Beanbag Throw
	Beanbag Toss
	Number Catch
	Space Demon
Subtraction:	Ten Litle Birds
	Take Away, Take Away
	Ten Little Chickadees
	Animal Catch
	Cheese and Mice
Multiplication:	Twice as Many
Division:	Triplet Tag
	Birds Fly South
	Birds Fly South (Variation)
Fractions:	Corner Spry
	End Ball
	Train Dodge
	Fraction Race
Decimals:	Roving Decimal Point
Measurement:	
Linear Measurement	
Liquid Measurement	Add-a-Jump Relay
Telling Time	Milkman Tag
Geometry:	Tick Tock
	Straight-Crooked Relay
	Around the Horn
	Run Circle Run
	Streets and Alleys
	Jump the Shot
	Triangle Run
	Geometric Figure Relay

Concept: Quantitative Aspects of Numbers and Numeral Recognition

Activity: Watch the Numbers

Write the numerals 1, 2, 3, 4, 5, 6 on large sheets of paper, one numeral per sheet. Write the numerals large enough so the children walking around the room can read them. The children start by walking around the room to music in single file. At any time the teacher may hold up one of the numerals. If the numeral is two, the children find partners and continue walking. If the numeral is three, the children walk in threes. Whenever a child does not secure a partner or becomes a part of the grouping, he goes to the sideline. When the next numeral appears, he rejoins the scramble to get into a correct formation.

Suggested Use: In this activity children are able to act out the quantitative aspects of numbers by forming appropriate-sized groups for the numeral called.

Concept: Quantitative Aspects of Numbers and Counting

Activity: Bee Sting

Three children are bees. They are in their hives marked in chalk on the activity area. The rest of the children are in the center of the designated activity area. The bees run out and try to catch (sting) the children. When a child is caught he must go to the bee's hive. When all the children are caught each bee counts those in his hive. Different children should have a chance to be bees.

Suggested Use: In this activity the children are provided another opportunity to practice counting. They can be helped to see the numbers of children caught by the bees in terms of being greater than and less than those caught by other bees. Children should note the quantitative aspects of numbers by counting and note that the numbers called represent objects, in this case children.

Concept: Quantitative Aspects of Numbers and Counting

Activity: Count and Go

The children line up on the long side of a rectangular hard surface court. There are parallel lines which are unequal distances apart drawn in chalk on the court. The teacher stands across from the children with number cards. The teacher holds up any card at random. (Numbers on the cards are from 1 to the total number in the group.) The children must count the lines as they run, skip and so on toward the teacher. (This should vary with the abilities of the group.) When the children get to the line that corresponds to the numeral on the card they should stop and stand still. The child who reaches the far side first is the winner.

Suggested Use: This activity reinforces counting as the children move forward the varying number of lines designated by the teacher. Another dimension to this activity would extend meaning to the concept of substraction. Directions could be presented such as plus two and minus three; the children would then proceed to carry out these directions in terms of moving forward and backward. The children should be helped to understand that the numeral 3 represents a group of three steps forward or backward.

Concept: Quantitative Aspects of Numbers and Counting
Activity: Muffin Man

The children stand in a circle with two children in the circle facing each other. While the first verse is sung, the children in the center stand still with hands on hips. When the second verse is sung, "Yes I know the Muffin Man, etc.," the two children clasp hands and skip around the outside of the circle, singing, Two of us know the Muffin Man, etc. At the end of the verse, these two children stand in front of two new partners and repeat the first and second verses. The second verse is now sung, "Four of us know the Muffin Man, etc." This procedure is repeated to eight, sixteen, etc., depending on the size of the group.

> Oh, do you know the Muffin Man,
> the Muffin Man, the Muffin Man?
> Oh, do you know the Muffin Man,
> who lives in Drury Lane?
> Yes, I know the Muffin Man,
> the Muffin Man, the Muffin Man.
> Yes, I know the Muffin Man
> who lives in Drury Lane.

Suggested Use: This activity provides children the opportunity to dramatize the grouping process in concrete number situations. Children might be helped between singing the verses to count out the numbers involved for the following verse. Number sentences might also be written on the chalkboard.

Concept: Quantitative Aspects of Numbers and Counting
Activity: Fish Net

The class is divided into two teams. One team is the net; the other is the fish. At the start the teams stand behind two goal lines at the opposite ends of the activity area, facing each other. When the teacher gives a signal, both teams run forward toward the center. The net tries to catch as many fish as possible by making a circle around them by holding hands. The fish try to get out of the opening before the net closes. They cannot go through the net by going under the arms of the children, but if the net breaks because the children let go of each other's hands, the fish can go through the opening until the hards are joined again. The fish are safe if they get to the opposite goal line without being caught in the net. When the net has made its circle, the number of fish inside are counted, and the score is recorded. The next time the teams change places.

Suggested Use: Children have the opportunity to count the number of fish caught each time. Counting in this situation acquires meaning for the children because they can relate number names to specific objects.

Concept: Quantitative Aspects of Numbers and Counting
Activity: Round Up

All but ten children of the group take places in a scattered formation on the activity area. The ten children join hands and are the round-up crew. The other children are the steers. On a signal, the round-up crew, with hands joined, chases the steers and attempts to surround one or more of them. To capture a steer, the two children of the round-up crew join hands. As the steers are captured, the children count the number aloud. They may have to stop and count each time another child is caught. When the tenth child is captured, they become the round-up crew, and the game continues.

Suggested Use: This activity enables children to apply number names in sequence to definite objects, in this case children. It provides practice in counting when the children check the number of steers caught up to that point in the activity until they reach the number 10.

Concept: Quantitative Aspects of Numbers and Counting
Activity: Chain Tag

One child is chosen as leader. The leader chooses another child to assist him, and the two join hands. They chase the other children, trying to tag one. When a child has been tagged, he takes his place between the two and the chain grows. The first two, the leader and his assistant, remain at the ends throughout the activity and are the only ones who can tag. When the chain surrounds a child, he may not break through the line or go under the hands. When the chain breaks, it must be reunited before the tagging begins again. The leader counts out loud every time he gets another child in his chain. The game ends when the chain has five or ten children. A new leader is chosen who in turn proceeds in the same manner.

Suggested Use: The children have practice in counting as each child is tagged. This activity helps to show the cardinal concept of numbers.

Concept: Quantitative Aspects of Numbers and Counting
Activity: Come With Me

The children stand close together in a circle. One child is *it*. *It* goes around the outside of the circle. *It* taps a child and says, Come with me. That child follows *it*. *It* continues in the same manner, tapping children who then follow *it* as he goes around the outside of the circle. At any time *it* may call, Go home! All the children following *it*, and *it* himself, run to find vacant places in the circle. The remaining child can be *it* for the next game. At the beginning the teacher has the children count how many there are at the start. *It* can count the children as he taps them. All the children also can be encouraged to count as *it* tags children. The number of children not tagged might also be counted.

Suggested Use: The children are able to practice counting varying-sized groups in this activity. By having *it* and all the children count as the children are tagged, each child is helped to see the number names related to specific objects.

Concept: Quantitative Aspects of Numbers and Counting
Activity: Ball Pass

The children are divided into two teams, and both teams form one single circle. If the group is large, the teacher may have two circles with two teams in each circle. The teacher gives directions for a ball to be passed or tossed from one child to another. The teacher calls, Pass the ball to the right, toss the ball to the left over two children. He varies the calls by the numbers and directions given. The game may be complicated by using more than one ball, the balls being of different sizes and weights. If a child drops a ball, a point is scored against his team. The team with the lowest score wins.

Suggested Use: The tasks in this activity provide children practice in relating numbers to specific quantities, which they act out, and in identifying right and left.

Concept: Quantitative Aspects of Numbers and Counting

Activity: Number Man

One child, the number man, faces the class standing on a line at the end of the activity area. Each child in the line is given a number by counting off. The number man calls out, "All numbers greater than _____." The children who have numbers greater than the one called must try to get to the other side without being tagged by the number man. The number man may also call out, "All numbers less than _____." Anyone who is tagged must help the number man tag the runners. Any child who runs out of turn is considered tagged.

Suggested Use: The children become familiar with counting and cardinal concepts through having to decide which numbers are greater than or less than.

Concept: Counting — In Multiples of 1's, 2's, 5's

Activity: Count, Move, and Stop

One child is *it*. He stands behind a finish line. All the other children are at a starting line that is drawn twenty-five to fifty feet away, parallel to the finish line. The children sit in a cross-legged sitting position, arms crossed on chest, at the starting line. The child who is *it* hides his eyes and counts to ten (or 20 or 100, depending upon the skills of the group) in any way he chooses, by ones, twos or fives. While *it* is counting, the players come to a standing position and move toward the finish line during the count. *It* must call the numbers loudly enough for all to hear. At the call of ten (or whatever number has been decided upon), *it* opens his eyes. All players must be seated cross-legged and with arms on chest, at the point to which they have advanced. Any child caught out of position must return to the starting line and begin again. The game continues in this manner until one child has crossed the finish line and is seated before *it* has completed the count. The first child over the line interrupts the count by calling, "Over!" All children return to the starting line, and the game begins again with this child as the new *it*.

Suggested Use: This activity provides the necessary repetition of counting by one's, two's and five's for each child since not only is *it* counting, but each child is counting in order to determine his movement forward.

Concept: Counting — in Multiples of 3's

Activity: Pick-Up Race

A number of wooden blocks (three or more for each child) are scattered over a large activity area. The children divide into several teams and take their places in rows behind a starting line. At the starting line there are circles drawn, one for each team. On a signal, the first child runs into the activity area and picks up one block, returns to the starting line, and places a block in his team's circle. He then goes back after a second block and returns it to the circle. He gets the third block and leaves the three blocks in a pile in the circle. The activity continues in this manner until each child on the team has collected and piled three blocks in the team's circle. The first team that completes the task wins.

Suggested Use: The children count out how many three's are necessary for each team and how many for all the teams together. Blocks may be counted in groups of three's for those children who have difficulty in identifying the quantity of blocks needed in order for them to see the number of blocks needed.

Concept: Counting — Forward and Backward

Activity: Pass Ball Relay

Children divide into teams. The team members line up one behind the other and close enough so they can easily pass a ball overhead to each other. On a signal, a ball is passed over each child's head to the end of the line. As the children pass the ball overhead they call out the numbers of their positions on the team as 1, 2, 3 until the ball reaches the end of the line. When the last child on the team receives the ball, he calls his number, then passes the ball forward again. The next to the last child calls out his number and continues passing the ball forward to the front of the team. For variation the ball may be passed in different ways — that is under the legs, alternating over and under. The winner is the first team to pass the ball forward and back with correct number-counting forward and backward.

Suggested Use: Children gain quickness in counting forward and backward in this activity. They are able to get a better understanding of ordinal numbers and their sequence. The teacher may start the counting at any number, depending on the skills of the group.

Concept: Counting — By 10's to 100

Activity: Red Light

Two lines are marked off thirty feet apart on the activity area. One child is *it*. The child who is *it* stands on one line. The remaining children are grouped at the other line. *It* turns his back to the children and counts loudly, "10, 20, 30, 40 ...... 100, red light!" The children advance toward him as he counts, but they must stop as he calls, "Red light!" As *it* calls, "Red light!" he turns, and if he sees a child moving, he sends the child back to the starting line. The object is to see which child can reach the goal line first.

Suggested Use: This activity gives both *it* and the other children the opportunity to practice counting by ten's, as they must count in order to know when to stop moving. With each child involved in counting, the activity provides the necessary repetition for all children.

Concept: Ordinal Numbers

Activity: Leader Ball

Two teams stand in circle formation. On a given signal, the leader of each team passes a ball to the player on his right, who passes it to the next player, and so on until it reaches the leader. The leader calls, First round! immediately and continues to pass the ball for the second round and third round. At the end of the third round the leader raises the ball to signify that his team has finished. A point is scored for the team finishing first.

Suggested Use: The time interval in counting by first round, second round, third round at the completion of passing the ball around the circle each turn helps to emphasize the ordinal concept of numbers. Children need to keep in mind the number to be called each time.

Concept: Ordinal Numbers

Activity: The Number Race

The class is divided into three teams of ten each. Each member of the teams is given a number from one to ten. They line up behind a starting line in correct numerical order. When the teacher gives a signal, the teams race to the finish line where the members sit down one behind the other in their proper order and in their proper groups. The first team finished scores a point. Number assignments should be frequently changed.

Suggested Use: Children are helped to note which numbers come before and after their number assignments. Changing numbers will help the children to develop greater facility with ordinal numbers.

Concept: Addition

Activity: Three Deep

The children stand by twos, one behind the other, in a circle. All face the center. A runner and chaser stand outside the circle. The chaser tries to tag the runner. In order to save himself, the runner may run around the circle and stand in front of one of the couples in the circle. This makes the group three deep, and the outside child in the group must now run. He is then chased and tries to save himself in the same way. The outside person in a group of three must always run. If the runner is tagged, he becomes the chaser and must turn and chase the new runner.

Suggested Use: The teacher assists the children in identifying groups of twos when the circle is formed for the game. When a runner stands in front of a group of two, the teacher assists the children in identifying that two and one make three.

Concept: Addition

Activity: Back to Back

The children stand back to back with arms interlocked at the elbows. The teacher calls for any size group. On a signal the children let go and must find a new partner if the teacher called for groups of two. Each time the teacher should have the children identify how many children must be added to one in order to make the size group that has been called. If the number called is larger than the group already formed, the teacher may ask how many children are needed to become the size group that has just been called for. Whatever the size group called for, the children must hook up, back to back, in that number. A time limit may be set. The children who are left over may rejoin the group each time a new set is called.

Suggested Use: In this activity the teacher can help the children to compare the sizes of the different groups. The teacher can help them act out the number of children to add to one or the existing group in order to form the next group called.

Concept: Addition

Activity: Beanbag Throw

Five large-mouth cans are tied together and are numbered from 1 to 5. The class is divided into two teams. A set of cans is required for each team. The teams stand in rows behind a line about ten feet from the targets. Each team member throws a beanbag, trying to get it in the number 5 can as it is worth the most points. Each child has three tries. At the end of his turn, each child adds up his score, and it is recorded for his team. When all the children have had their turns, they add the scores to find which team has the most points.

Suggested Use: An activity of this type stimulates interest in arithmetic practice. This activity may be done with higher numbers as the children progress. Children who are having difficulty in adding may be helped by the teacher to count out their scores.

Concept: Addition (1 — 10)

Activity: Beanbag Toss

A board is made three or four feet square with a small eight inch circle cut out in the center of the square. A child standing ten feet from the board tosses five beanbags, one at a time, at the board. If he hits the square he scores one point and three points if the beanbag goes through the hole in the center. The child totals his score and records it.

Suggested Use: This activity enables the children to use their addition facts in an interesting and motivating situation in their totaling of their scores.

Concept: Addition (1 — 10)

Activity: Number Catch

Every child is given a number from 1 to 10. The teacher calls "two plus two" or "six plus one," and tosses the ball into the air. Any child whose number happens to be the sum of the numbers called can catch the ball. The other children run away as fast as they can until the child catches the ball and calls, "Stop!" At that time all the children must stop where they are and remain standing in place. The child with the ball may take three long running strides in any direction toward the children. If he succeeds, the child who is hit has a point scored against him. The game continues with the teacher calling out another addition problem. The children with the lowest number of points are the winners.

Suggested Use: Follows this section of activities for reinforcement of addition facts inasmuch as the application is the same.

Concept: Addition (1 — 10)

Activity: Space Demon

There are twenty-one children with ten on each team and a Space Demon. The two teams line up facing each other about twenty feet apart. The distance between the two teams represents space. Each team counts off so each member is assigned a number. The teacher calls out an addition problem whose sum will not be greater than 10. The children representing the parts of the problem (the addends) as well as the children representing the answer or sum from each team try to exchange places before the space demon tags one of them. If a child is tagged, his team gets one point. The team with the lowest score within a set time wins.

Suggested Use: Follows this section of activities for reinforcement of addition facts.

Concept: Subtraction

Activity: Ten Little Birds

The children form a circle. Ten children are selected for the birds, and they count off from 1 to 10. They go into the center of the circle and stand in a line within the circle. When the verses are sung, the child in the center with the number being repeated flies back to his original position in the circle formed by the children. This is repeated until all the birds have moved back to the circle with the other children. The song may be sung again with other children selected to be birds.

> Ten little birds sitting on a line
> One flew away and then there were nine.
>
> Nine little birds sitting up straight,
> One fell down and then there were eight.
>
> Eight little birds looking up to heaven,
> One went away and then there were seven.

Seven little birds picking up sticks,
One flew away and then there were six.

Six little birds sitting on a hive,
One got stung and then there were five.

Five little birds peeping through a door,
One went in and then there were four.

Four little birds sitting in a tree,
One fell down and then there were three.

Three little birds looking straight at you,
One went home and then there were two.

Two little birds sitting in the sun,
One went home and then there was one.

One little bird left all alone,
He flew away and then there were none.

Suggested Use: In this activity, children are able to act out the concept of subtraction. The children can understand more readily by seeing the group grow smaller each time one is taken away.
Concept: Subtraction
Activity: Take Away, Take Away

The children stand in a circle. One child is *it*. He walks around inside the circle. As the children sing the following song, to the tune of "Twinkle Twinkle Little Star," they act out the words of the song.

Take away, take away, take away one.
Come with me and have some fun.

Take away, take away, take away two.
Come with me, oh yes please do.

Take away, take away, take away three.
All please come and skip with me.

It taps one child. This child follows behind *it*. *It* then taps a

second and third child. At the end of the song all three children try
to get back to their places in the circle. *It* also tries to get into one
of the vacant places. The remaining child becomes *it* for the next
time.

Suggested Use: This activity enables children to see demonstrated
the concept of subtraction. The teacher may have the children
identify how many children are left each time *it* takes away one
child.

Concept: Subtraction

Activity: Ten Little Chickadees

Groups of ten children form lines, facing forward. The
children in each line count off 1 to 10 from left to right. As the
verses are sung, the child with that number sits down.

Ten little chickadees standing in a line,
One flew away and now there are nine.

Nine little chickadees standing very straight,
One flew away and now there are eight.

Eight little chickadees looking up to heaven,
One flew away and now there are seven.

Seven little chickadees build a nest of sticks,
One flew away and now there are six.

Six little chickadees looking much alive,
One flew away and now there are five.

Five little chickadees pecking at the door,
One flew away and now there are four.

Four little chickadees all afraid of me,
One flew away and now there are three.

Three little chickadees don't know what to do,
One flew away and now there are two.

Two little chickadees looking at the sun,

One flew away and now there is one.

One little chickadee hopping on the ground,
He flew away and now none are around.

Suggested Use: Children are able to visualize the subtraction process in this activity. The teacher may stop the song at any point and have the children identify the subtraction fact appropriate for that particular verse. After the song the teacher might have the children write the different number sentences.

Concept: Subtraction
Activity: Animal Catch

Two parallel lines about twenty feet apart are marked off. One child, the animal catcher, stands in the center area between the two lines. On one of the lines, the other children form in groups of four (or five, six, etc.) facing the animal catcher. Each group selects the name of an animal such as bear, elephant, camel or tiger. The animal catcher calls the name of one group of animals. These children try to run to the opposite line without being tagged by the animal catcher. If so, they remain as animals. Those children who are caught help the animal catcher to tag members of the other animal groups when called.

Suggested Use: The teacher helps the children to identify groups of four or whatever size group is selected. At intervals during the activity, the teacher has the opportunity to develop the meaning of subtraction by asking such questions as, "How many horses were caught?," "How many did we start with?," "How many were left?" Children can be helped to count out the answers if necessary.

Concept: Subtraction
Activity: Cheese and Mice

A round mousetrap is formed by the children standing in a circle. In the center of the mousetrap is placed the cheese (a ball or some other object). The children are each assigned numbers (0, 1, 2, up to 10). Several children can be assigned to each number. When the teacher calls a number from 0 to 10, all the children with the number that represents the difference or remainder of the number called from 10 leave their places in the circle, run around the outside of the circle, then return to their original places (hole in the trap). They then run into the circle to get the cheese. The first child to get the cheese is the winning mouse. The teacher must check to see that the children with the correct number for the answer to the problem were the mice who ran to get the cheese. Only a child with the correct number can win.

Suggested Use: In this activity the children are provided opportunity for practice in subtraction facts whose differences is less than 10. Speed and accuracy can be developed. The teacher may assign other numbers and call out more difficult problems according to the skills of the group. This activity can be adapted to addition, multiplication and division.

Concept: Multiplication by 2's
Activity: Twice as Many

The children stand on a line near the end of the activity area and face the caller. The caller stands at the finish line some twenty-five to fifty feet away and gives directions as, Take two hops. Now take twice as many. Take three small steps. Now take twice as many.

Directions are varied in number and type of movement. Each direction is followed by, "Now take twice as many." The first child to reach the finish line calls out, "Twice as many!" and everyone runs back to the starting line. The caller tags all those he can before they reach the starting line. All those tagged help the caller the next time.

Suggested Use: Children are able to apply their *multiplication-by-two* facts to a highly motivating activity. The teacher may check each time a new direction is given to be sure the children have multiplied by two accurately and have the correct answer. This activity encourages children to respond quickly to multiplication facts. Those children who are having difficulty may be helped by the teacher to act out the multiplication fact called for.

Concept: Division
Activity: Triplet Tag

The children form groups of three with hands joined. As the groups are formed the teacher should point out that the total number of children to be divided is the *dividend,* the group size of three children is the *divisor,* and the resulting number of groups is the *quotient.* If the whole groups cannot be divided equally, the children will see that there are some left over or a *remainder*. The groups stand scattered about the activity area. One groups is *it* and carries a red cloth. The group that is *it* tries to tag another group of three. Hands must be joined at all times. When a group is tagged it is given the red cloth, and the game continues.

Suggested Use: The children have the opportunity to act out the division process in this activity. The children can readily see the quotient by counting the groups.

Concept: Division — The Effect of Decreasing or Increasing the Divisor on the Quotient When the Dividend Remains the Same

Activity: Birds Fly South

Play begins with the entire class distributed randomly behind a starting line. The entire class represents the dividend. A caller gives the signal to play by calling, Birds fly south in flocks of six (or the highest number that will be used to divide the number, the divisor). The class runs to another line that has been designated as South. At this point the children should be grouped in sixes. After observing the number of flocks (the quotient), the remainders become hawks who take their places between the two lines. Then with the call, "Scatter, the hawks are coming!" the children run back to the other line with the hawks attempting to tag them. Note is taken of who is tagged. Play continues with the entire class taking its place behind the starting line. The caller then uses the lowest number for the call. If six was used first, five would be called next, "Birds fly south in flocks of five." This continues until the smallest groups can be made which would be two. Each time the children should observe the number of flocks (the quotient).

To score the game, each child would begin with a score equivalent to the number which is called first — that is, in this case, the number six. If he is tagged, his score increases by one point.

Suggested Use: At the end of the game, the class should evaluate the arithmetic learning involved by noting that when the total number of children remained the same (dividend) and the size of the flocks (divisor) decreased, the number of flocks (quotient) increased. After this pattern has been established, the numbers called can be reversed, beginning with the smallest divisor and working up to the highest divisor to be used. Here the converse of the previous understanding can be developed.

Concept: Division — The Effect of Decreasing or Increasing the Dividend on the Quotient When the Divisor Remains the Same
Activity: Birds Fly South (Variation)

Starting with the entire class on the starting line, at the signal, "Birds fly south in flocks of six" (or the highest number that would be used to divide the number), the class runs to the line designated as South. At this point they should group by sixes or whatever the divisor. After observing the quotient in terms of the number of *flocks,* the remainders become hawks who take their place between the two lines. Then, with the call, "Scatter, the hawks are coming!" the children ungroup and run back to the other line with the hawks attempting to tag them. All children caught and hawks retire to a *hawks' nest.* A point is scored by the individuals left when the total can no longer be divided into the groups originally established as the divisor.

Suggested Use: The change in total number of children at the starting line (dividend) each time is noted, and play continues in like manner with emphasis put on the number of flocks or groups that is the outcome when the dividend has been reduced.

Concept: Fractions — Numerator and Demoninator
Activity: Corner Spry

In a rectangular activity area, a circle about ten feet in diameter is marked in the center. There are four equal teams, and a captain for each team is chosen. One team is in each corner of the playing area while the four captains take their places inside the circle. Each captain has a ball. There is a caller assigned, and there may be a scorer. Each team member represents one part of the total number on the team — that is he may represent one third, one fourth or one eighth of the team. The caller calls different fractions (involving thirds, fourths or eighths, depending on the total number of children on the teams) in any order. When the caller calls a fraction, that number of each team must take a squatting position. The captain of each team will then pass and receive the ball with each member of his team remaining standing. The first one finished with this exchange without dropping the ball scores a point, and another fraction is called.

Suggested Use: Children should be helped to note that the number of children who squat (numerator) represent the number of parts of the total number of units (denominator) being used.

Concept: Fractions

Activity: End Ball

An activity area twenty-five by fifty feet is marked off. The area is then divided by lines so that four lines (including the end lines) are equidistant from each other about twelve feet apart. The class is divided into two teams. Each team is then divided into two groups. The groups from each team take places along the four lines so they alternate with the groups of the other team. The object of the activity is for each team to try to throw the ball over the heads of the opposing team. Points are scored when the ball is caught by the opposing team as it is thrown over their heads. The team with the highest score within a given time limit wins.

Suggested Use: The children are helped to find one half of the class to make up the two teams. They then find one half of each team to form the two groups within each team. It can be brought out that each group represents one fourth of the total class number. It can also be brought out that to divide the class into fourths, the total number of the class could have been divided by four. Children can then be encouraged to find other parts, divisions or fractions of other size groups.

Concept: Subtraction of Fractions

Activity: Train Dodge

The class forms a circle with four children in the center. The children in the center hold each other about the waist, thus making a train, standing one behind the other. The object of the game is to tag the *caboose* or last child. One or more rubber inflated balls may be used to try to hit the caboose. As the caboose is hit, he can temporarily wait outside the circle. The game continues until all four children of the train have been hit. At the outset the teacher establishes the concept that the four children within the circle make up the *whole* train, that each child is one part, one fourth of the whole train. As each child is hit and moves to the outside of the circle, a brief pause is taken to ascertain that one fourth of the train is now uncoupled and waiting outside, and three fourths of the cars remain coupled together and in the game.

When the next child is hit, then two fourths are in and two fourths are out. Finally, the whole train is assembled outside the circle and is now in the roundhouse. A new train is then formed with another group of four children.

Suggested Use: This activity provides a dramatic means of presenting subtraction of fractions. Midway through the activity, the teacher might help the children to note two fourths are one half the train, and that an equal number of cars are inside and outside the circle.

Concept: Fractions

Activity: Fraction Race

The class is divided into a number of teams. The members of each team taking a sitting position, one behind the other, a specified distance from a goal line. Starting with the first child on the teams, the children are assigned numbers starting with the number 1. The teacher calls out a fraction of a number. The children whose number is the answer, stand, run to the goal line, and return to their original sitting position. If the teacher calls out, "one fourth of eight!" all the number 2's would run. Similarly, if the teacher calls, "one third of fifteen!" all the number 5's would run. The first child back scores five points for his team, the second child back scores three points, and the last child scores one point. The team with the highest score wins.

Suggested Use: In this activity the children are called upon to develop quickness in working out fractions of whole numbers. When necessary, children can work out their problem by counting to help them see the answer.

Concept: Decimals

Activity: Roving Decimal Point

Children line up in teams with about five children to a team. A team captain stands in front of each team ready to record scores. A ball, representing the decimal point, is given to the first child on each team. On a given signal, the ball is bounced or passed from child to child up the line, then back again. When the stop signal is given, the decimal point (the ball) stops and is put to the left of the child last holding the ball. Each child then has to tell what place (fraction denominator) he represents. A point is given for each correct answer. If the ball is dropped, it must be taken to the first child on the team and started down the line again. When everyone has learned the value of each place to the right of the decimal point, the children might be assigned numbers, as the activity proceeds as before except this time the captain is required to read the decimal number they represent in order to score. The captain can join the line, and the last child becomes captain after each scoring until each has a turn at being captain. The team having the highest score wins.

Suggested Use: This activity can be used in developing understanding and skill in reading decimal numbers.

Concept: Linear Measurement

Activity: Add-a-Jump Relay

Teams form single lines. The first child of each team moves up to a starting line in front of his team and jumps as far as he can. This distance is marked. The second child walks to this mark and jumps as far as he can. This continues until each child on the teams has jumped. The team covering the greatest distance is declared the winner.

Suggested Use: When children are working with linear measures, this relay helps them to be able to measure distances and to gain understanding of how to add, subtract and compare distance. After each child has had his turn, he can measure the distance of his jump and record it in feet and inches. Children can be assigned to measure the total distance jumped by each team. When the children return to the classroom, they can use these figures to find the average distance jumped, to compare team or individual records, and to add individual distances together and check totals with the recorded team distance. Practice with changing measures to smaller or larger units is provided.

Concept: Liquid Measurement — Pints and Quarts

Activity: Milkman Tag

Two teams of three milkmen are selected and given milk truck bases (a tree for instance). One team might be called chocolate, the other white. The remaining children are called pints. On a given signal, one milkman from each team tries to tag any one of the pints. When he tags one, they both go to the milk truck, and another milkman goes after a pint. A goal may be set as to the number of pints needed for a team to win. The teacher can set a goal of so many quarts to be gained in order to win. The children must then figure out how many pints will be needed to make the necessary number of quarts. They may multiply the number of quarts by two or they may pair off the pints and add to determine the number needed for the specified number of quarts.

Suggested Use: Children are provided a highly motivating activity to work with pints and quarts and their equivalents. Children can count the number of pints caught by each team and group them to figure out if they have the correct number of quarts.

Concept: Telling Time

Activity: Tick Tock

The class forms a circle that represents a clock. Two children are runners and are called hour and minute. The children chant, "What time is it?" Minute then chooses the hour and calls it out (six o'clock). Hour and minute must stand still while the children in the circle call, "One o'clock, two o'clock, three o'clock . . . six o'clock" (or whatever time has been chosen). When the children get to the chosen hour, the chase begins. Hour chases minute clockwise around the outside of the circle. If hour can catch minute before the children in the circle once again call out "One o'clock, two o'clock . . . six o'clock" (the same hour as counted the first time), he chooses another child to become hour. The game can also be played counting by half hours.

Suggested Use: Children not only get practice in calling the hours, but they develop an understanding of the concept of the term *clockwise*.

Concept: Telling Time

Activity: Five-Minute Relay

The class is divided into relay teams. A cardboard clock with movable hands is set up for each team at the front of the room. The clocks are set for any given time. Each clock may be set at a different time so the teams cannot copy each other. The teams are in relay formation a specified distance from the clocks. On a signal, the first child on each team begins the relay by running forward and moves the minute hand ahead by five minutes and writes down the next time on the board. As soon as this child is past the first child on his team when he moves forward to the clock, the team moves back leaving a space for the first child up at the front of the team's line. As soon as the first child returns, he raises his hand, and the last child on the team proceeds. He moves the minute hand ahead five minutes and writes down the time. The first team whose runners all finish setting the clock and writing down the time correctly wins.

Suggested Use: In this activity the children are provided the repetition necessary for learning to tell time quickly and accurately. This activity helps to reinforce the skills previously presented in situations that are highly motivating.

Concept: Geometry — The Shortest Distance Between Two Points Is a Straight Line

Activity: Straight-Crooked Relay

The class is divided into four teams. In the relay, one team runs directly between two points while the second team has an additional place to tag between the two points that is not in direct line with the other points. Teams should be switched so that they alternate having to run the crooked route.

Suggested Use: The children can note that it takes less time to move between two points by following a straight line than by following a crooked line because a straight line is the shortest distance. The children can measure the distance of the straight and crooked lines between the two points that are equidistant for the two teams. To account for individual differences of children the teacher might make sure that both slow and fast runners are assigned to each team.

Concept: Geometry — The Meaning of Perimeter; The Shortest Distance Between Two Points is a Straight Line

Activity: Around the Horn

A small playing area is set up similar to a baseball diamond with a home plate and three bases. The team in the field has a catcher on home plate and two fielders on each of the bases. The runners of the other team stand in a file at home plate. The catcher has the ball. The object is for the catcher and fielders, on a signal, to relay the ball around the bases and back to home plate *twice* before the runner at home plate can run around, tag each base and proceed to home plate *once*. At the bases the fielders take turns. One takes the first throw, the other the second. The team up to the plate scores a point if it reaches home plate before the ball.

Suggested Use: The distance around the bases is described as the perimeter of the field. Each runner is told he must run the perimeter of the field, and the team in the field is told that the ball must go twice around the perimeter of the field. The children learn that a wild throw which is not in a straight line to the other player takes longer to get to the next base.

Concept: Geometry — A Circle is a Simple Closed Curve Surrounding a Closed Region

Activity: Run, Circle, Run

The class forms a circle by holding hands and facing inward. Depending on the size of the group, the children count off by two's or three's for small groups, or four's, five's or six's for large groups around thirty. The teacher calls one of the assigned numbers. All the children with that number start running around the circle; each runner tries to tag one or more children running ahead of him. As successful runners reach their starting point without being tagged, they stop. Runners who are tagged go to the center of the circle. Another number is called, and the same procedure is followed. This is continued until all have been called. Reform the circle, assign new numbers to the children, and repeat. As the number of children decreases, a circle may be drawn on the ground which they must stay out of when running around the circle to their places.

Suggested Use: The children should be helped to note that when they form a circle by holding hands they make a continuous, simple, closed curve. As they play the game they should observe what happens when segments break off. They also see how the curve surrounds a region, because the children who are standing in the center represent points in space within the region.

Concept: Geometry — Parallel Lines and Right Angles

Activity: Streets and Alleys

The children divide into three or more parallel lines with at least three feet between children in each direction. A runner and chaser are chosen. The children all face the same direction and join hands with those on each side forming streets between the rows. Dropping hands, the children make a quarter turn and join hands again and form alleys. The chaser tries to tag the runner going up and down the streets or alleys, but not breaking through or going under arms. The teacher aids the runner by calling streets or alleys at the proper time. At this signal the children drop hands, turn and grasp hands in the opposite direction, thus blocking the passage of the chaser. When caught, the runner and chaser select two others to take their places. If the runner is not caught within a reasonable amount of time, a new runner and chaser can be selected.

Suggested Use: The children should be helped to note that the streets and alleys represent parallel lines that, no matter how far they are extended, they will not meet. When the teacher calls alleys, and the children make a quarter turn, the children should note that they have made a right-angle turn, and represent the concept of right angles.

Concept: Geometry — Radius of a Circle
Activity: Jump the Shot

The children make a circle in groups of eight or ten, facing the center. One child stands in the center of the circle with a bean bag tied to the end of a rope. The center child swings the rope around in a large circle low enough to the ground in order for the bean bag to pass under the feet of those in the circle. The children in the circle attempt to jump over the bean bag as it passes beneath their feet. When the rope or bean bag touches a child, it is a point against him. The child with the lowest score wins at the end of a period of one or two minutes. The child in the center may then exchange places.

Suggested Use: Children note that the radius of the circle is the length of the rope to which the beanbag is tied, and is the distance from the center of the circle to the edge of the circle where the children stand. The teacher may draw a circle in order for the children to see this more clearly. The children can be helped to see the radius is the same from any part of the edge of the circle to the center.

Concept: Geometric Forms — Triangle
Activity: Triangle Run

A large triangle is marked off with a base at each corner. Three equal-sized teams are formed. One team stands behind each base. On a signal, the first child of each team leaves his base and runs to his right around the triangle, touching each base on the way. When he returns to his base, the next child on his team does the same. The runners may pass each other, but they must touch each base as they run. The first team back in its original place wins. *Suggested Use:* This activity helps to show the shape of the triangle and demonstrates the concept of its perimeter. Children should note that the triangle must have three angles (where the bases are). At different times different shape triangles may be marked off for the activity to demonstrate that the essence of the triangle is found in its three angles and three sides, not its shape.

Concept: Geometric Figures

Activity: Geometric Figure Relay

Two lines are drawn about thirty feet apart on the activity area. The class is divided into two teams. Both teams stand behind one of the lines. The teacher calls out the name of a geometric figure. The teams run across to the opposite line to form the figure. The team that forms the figure correctly first wins a point. The teams then line up behind that line, and when the teacher calls another figure, they run to the opposite line and again form the figure the teacher has called. The geometric figures will be those that the children have been working with including the circle, square, rectangle and the triangle.

Suggested Use: Children can gain the understanding of different geometric figures by acting out their shapes in an interesting activity.

CHAPTER SEVEN

LEARNING ABOUT SCIENCE
THROUGH MOTOR ACTIVITY

THE opportunities for science experiences through motor activity are so numerous that it is difficult to visualize a motor oriented experience that is not related to science in some way. Indeed, the possibilities for a better understanding of science and the application of science principles in motor activities are almost unlimited. Yet teachers are sometimes oblivious to many of these possibilities. Indicative of this paradoxical situation is the following anedote related by Herrick many years ago.[1]

One cold day when the sixth graders came in from an outdoor play period several children were discussing what could be the matter with their large rubber and soccer balls. When they took them from the cupboard they seemed to be blown up hard enough, but after being used on the playground for a short period of time they were too soft. The teacher ended the conversation by saying, "Play period is over. Put the balls away, and get ready for science class. We are starting our unit on air today."

If children are to be provided with learning experiences in science that involve the study of problems that are of real concern in their lives, teachers might well be on the alert for those things of interest to pupils in the daily school situation.

Although the main purpose of this chapter is to deal with *specific* ways to learn about science through motor activity, some mention should be made about how this can occur *generally*.

GENERAL WAYS OF USING MOTOR ACTIVITIES
IN TEACHING ABOUT SCIENCE

The following generalized list is submitted to give the reader an

---

[1]Virgil E. Herrick, *Issues in Elementary Education*. Minneapolis, Burgess Publishing Company, 1952, p. 155.

idea of some of the possible ways in which opportunities for science experiences might be utilized through various kinds of motor activities.

1. The physical principle of *equilibrium* or state of balance is one that is involved in many motor activities. This is particularly true of *stunt* activities in which balance is so important to proficient performance.

2. *Motion* is obviously the basis for all motor activities. Consequently, there is opportunity to relate laws of motion, at least in an elementary way, to movement experiences of children.

3. Children may perhaps understand better the application of *force* when it is thought of in terms of hitting a ball with a bat or in tussling with an opponent in a combative stunt.

4. *Friction* may be better understood by the use of a rubber-soled gym shoe on a hard-surfaced playing area.

5. Throwing or batting a ball against the wind can show how *air friction* reduces the speed of flying objects.

6. Accompaniment for rhythmic activities such as the drum, piano and recordings help children to learn that *sounds* differ from one another in pitch, volume and quality.

7. The fact that *force of gravitation* tends to pull heavier-than-air objects earthward may be better understood when the child finds that he must aim above a target at certain distances.

8. Ball-bouncing presents a desirable opportunity for a better understanding of *air pressure*.

9. *Weather* might be better understood on those days when it is too inclement to go outside to the activity area. In this same connection, weather and climate can be considered with regard to the various sport seasons — that is baseball in spring and summer, and games that are suited to winter play and cold climates.

It should be understood that the above represent just a partial list of such possibilities, and a person with just a little ingenuity could expand it to a much greater length.

THE SCIENCE MOTOR ACTIVITY STORY

It might be well at the outset of this discussion to take into account some of the prevailing ideas with reference to *integrating* science and reading.

It has been suggested by many that interest in science can provide motivation for a desire to read. The validity of this notion is inherent in the current national interest in the right to read. Moreover, it is common knowledge that in some elementary schools, focus has been placed on reading to the extent that teaching in other subject areas is being oriented to improvement in reading.

Another point of view tends to hold that whatever success a child has in science should be dependent upon his ability in the area of science. Some elementary school specialists have expressed it as follows,

> Without denying the heavy reliance which all intellectual activities must have upon language skills, we wish to remind you of the equally desirable goal of permitting the child who lacks language skills to find other success in the classroom. Science is one of the subjects which *can* be studied without undue emphasis upon language. In this connection, we discourage the practice of requiring the mastery of an extensive science vocabulary except that needed to communicate within the classroom.[2]

It should be pointed out that the preceding schools of thought are not necessarily diametrically opposed. Thus, there is allowance for a degree of reliance of science and reading upon each other.

Early attempts to develop science motor activity stories were patterned after the original procedure used in providing for motor-oriented reading content discussed in *Chapter Five* — that is several stories were written around certain kinds of motor activities, the only difference being that the content also involved reference to science experiences. These stories were tried out in a number of situations. It soon became apparent, as was the case in the mathematics motor activity story, that with some children the development of science concepts in a story was too difficult. The reason for this appeared to be that certain children could not

---

[2]Wm. Vernon Hicks et al., *The New Elementary School Curriculum*. New York, Van Nostrand Reinhold Company, 1970, p. 113.

handle both the task of reading while at the same time developing an understanding of the science aspect of the story. It was then decided that since *listening* is a first step in learning to read, auditory input should be utilized. This procedure involved having children listen to a story, perform the activity and simultaneously try to develop the science concept that was inherent in the story. When it appeared desirable this process was extended by having the children read the story after having engaged in the activity.

The following example of a science motor activity story presented here is taken from *Learning to Listen and Read Through Movement* by the present author and referred to in *Chapter Five*. This book contains over sixty stories about such motor activities as games, rhythms and stunts. Guidelines for teachers are presented for use of the materials. The content of the stories involves various curriculum areas in different ways, and the example that follows may be said to have a science flavor.

This example concerns the game Shadow Tag which is played in the following manner: The players are dispersed over the activity area with one person designated as *it*. If *it* can step on or get into the shadow of another player, that player becomes *it*. A player can keep from being tagged by getting into the shade or by moving in such a way that *it* finds it difficult to step on his shadow. The story about this game is The Shadow Game.

The Shadow Game

Have you ever watched shadows?

When do you see your shadow?

What can your shadow do?

Here is a game to play with shadows.

You can play it with one or more children.

You can be *it*.

Tell your friends to run around,
  so you can not step on their shadow.

When you step on a shadow,
  that child becomes *it*.

You join the other players.

Could you step on someone's shadow?

In one specific situation at first grade level this story was used to introduce the concept *shadows are formed by sun shining on various objects*. Following this a definition of a shadow was given. A discussion led the class to see how shadows are made as well as why they move. The class then went outside the room to the hardtop area where many kinds of shadows were observed. Since each child had a shadow it was decided to put them to use in playing the game.

In evaluating the experience, the teacher felt that the children saw how the sun causes shadows. By playing the game at different times during the day they also observed that the length of the shadow varied with the time of day. It was generalized that the story and the participation in the activity proved very good for illustrating shadows.

It is highly recommended by the author that teachers draw upon their own ingenuity and creativeness to prepare science motor-oriented stories, instructions for which have been given in a previous chapter.

SELECTED MOTOR ACTIVITIES TO
DEVELOP SCIENCE CONCEPTS

The following is a summary of motor activities along with the inherent science concepts which are explained in detail in the ensuing section of the chapter. The activities are grouped arbitrarily according to certain areas of study. Descriptions of the activities along with suggestions for use follow the summary.

Concept	Activity
The Universe and Earth:	
Planet's Orbit Around the Sun	Planet Ball
Earth's Orbit Around the Sun	Earth's Orbit Relay
Eclipse of the Moon	Eclipse Tag
Force of Gravity	Catch the Cane
Earth's Atmoshpere	Balloon Throw
	Air Lift
	Water Cycle Relay
Earth's Surface:	Zig Zag Run
Conditions of Life	
Variety of Life	
	Squirrels in Trees
	Animal Relay
	Snail
	Flowers and Wind

Interdependence of Life	Fox and Geese
	Spider and Flies
	Herds and Flocks
	Fox and Sheep
Chemical and Physical Changes:	Molecule Ball
	Molecule Pass
	Boiling Water
	Tag and Stoop
	Oxygen and Fuel
Light	Light Bounce
	Heat and Light
	Spectrum Relay
Energy:	
Machines	Pin Guard
	Hot Potato
	Net Ball
Electricity	Electric Ball
	Current Relay
	Lightning Relay
	Keep Away
Magnetism	Link Tag
	Hook-On Tag
	North and South
	Magnet, Magnet
Sound	Stoop Tag

The Universe and Earth

Concept: Planets' Orbit Around the Sun
Activity: Planet Ball

The children form a single circle and count off by two's. The number 1's step forward, turn, and face the number 2's. The larger circle should be about four feet outside the inner circle. Two children, designated as team captains, stand opposite each other in the circle. The teacher stands in the center of the circle and represents the sun. Each captain has a ball that his team identifies as a planet. On a signal from the teacher, each ball is passed counterclockwise to each team member until it travels all the way around the circle and back to the captain. Any child who is responsible for the ball striking the floor, either through a poor throw or a failure to catch the ball, has to recover the ball. As both circles pass the balls simultaneously, the time is kept and recorded. The group that passes the ball around their circle first wins or scores a point. Groups should exchange positions every several rounds.

Suggested Use: Prior to playing the game, the children should note the balls being passed around are the planets and that they are revolving around the sun represented by the teacher. They should be helped to identify the balls that are being passed counterclockwise because that is the direction the planets orbit the sun. In using this activity to illustrate the orbits of planets, it should be stressed that the path or orbit of the ball should be unbroken or uninterrupted. It should also be noted that each completed orbit was done with different amounts of time for each circle, and that the inner circle tended to take less time to pass the ball around. Children can be encouraged to find out the differences in the orbits of the planets as well as the varying lengths of times of these orbits.

Concept: Earth's Orbit Around the Sun

Activity: Earth's Orbit Relay

The children are arranged in two circles, each circle facing in. A captain is selected for each team, and they stand ready with balls in their hands. On a signal, each captain starts his team's ball around by passing to the child on his right. Upon receiving the ball, each child spins around and passes the ball on to the next child on the right. As the ball makes a complete circuit back to the captain, he calls, "One!" The second time around he calls, "Two!" This procedure is repeated until the first team to pass the ball around the circle five times wins.

Suggested Use: In this activity the children need to be helped to see they are dramatizing the way the earth revolves around the sun. The entire circle becomes the complete orbit of the earth. The ball represents the earth, and as it is passed from one child to another, they can see how the earth revolves around the sun. Also, since each child must spin around with the ball before passing it on, the concept of the earth's rotation on its axis may be shown. The children must always turn and pass counterclockwise since that is the direction of the earth's orbit.

Concept: The Turning of the Earth on Its Axis Causes Day and Night

Activity: Night and Day

The children stand in a circle holding hands. One child in the center of the circle represents the earth. As the children hold hands, they chant,

Illery, dillery, daxis,
The earth turns on its axis.
Isham, bisham bay,
It turns from night to day.

While the children are chanting, earth closes his eyes and turns slowly with one hand pointing towards the circle of children. As he rotates slowly with eyes closed (night), he continues to point with his hand. At the word *day* he stops and opens his eyes (day). Earth then runs after the child to whom he is pointing at the word *day*; they run around the outside of the circle until he catches him. When the child is caught, he becomes the new earth. The original earth joins the circle, and the game continues. It might be advisable to use a blindfold that the child can slip off at the end of the verse.

Suggested Use: The child in the center becomes the rotating earth. When his eyes are closed it becomes night, and when his eyes are open it becomes day. The children might be encouraged to think of the child being pointed to as the sun since it is day when the eyes are opened, and the sun causes day.

Concept: Eclipse of the Moon
Activity: Eclipse Tag

The children are grouped by couples facing each other. The couples are scattered in any way about the activity area. One child is chosen for the runner and is called the earth. Another child is the chaser. On a signal, the chaser tries to tag earth. Earth is safe from being tagged when he runs and steps between two children who make up a couple. When earth steps between the two children he calls out, "Eclipse!" The chaser must then chase the child in the couple toward whom earth turns his back. If the chaser is able to tag earth, they exchange places.

Suggested Use: This activity enables children to dramatize the concept of an eclipse of the moon so that they can see what occurs. The children should be helped to identify that when earth steps between two children, the one he faces is the moon and his back is turned to the sun, and that the earth's shadow covers the moon.

Concept: Force of Gravity
Activity: Catch the Cane

The children are arranged in a circle, facing in. Each child is given a number. One child becomes *it* and stands in the center of the circle. He holds a stick or bat upright and balances it by putting his finger on the top of it. *It* calls one of the numbers assigned to the children in the circle. At the same time, he lets go of the stick. The child whose number is called dashes to get the stick before it falls to the ground. *It* dashes to the place occupied by the child whose number was called. If the child gets the stick in time then he returns to his place in the circle, and *it* holds the stick again. After the children have learned the game, several circles can be formed to provide active participation for more children. The teacher can provide for individual differences of poor performers by making the circle smaller.

Suggested Use: The stick in this game represents the object which is being acted upon by the force of gravity. Every time *it* lets go of the stick, the stick begins to fall to the ground. This demonstrates the concept of the force of gravity to children. They may be helped to note that they must move faster than the force of gravity in order to catch the stick before it falls to the ground.

Concept: Force of Gravity

Activity: Jump the Shot

The children form a circle with one child in the center. The center child has a length of rope with a beanbag attached to one end. He holds the rope at the other end and swings the rope around close to the ground. The children in the circle must jump over the rope to keep from being hit. Any child who fails to jump and is hit receives a point against him. The child with the least number of points at the end of the game is the winner.

Suggested Use: The game is played in small groups, and each child should have a turn to be in the center and swing the rope. The teacher might ask the children what they felt on the other end of the rope as they swung it around — that is if they felt a pull. The teacher can ask what would happen if the rope broke or if they let go of their end. This can be demonstrated. Further questions can lead to what kept the rope and beanbag from flying off during the game, what the inward pull was on the rope that kept the beanbag moving in a circular pattern. The teacher might also relate this to the manner planets travel in a circular orbit around the sun and the moon circles the earth because of gravitational force.

Concept: Gravitational Pull — of Tides, Planets

Activity: Planet Pull (Tide Pull)

The children are divided into two teams. One can be named earth, and the other, moon. The first child on each team kneels down on all fours, facing a member of the other team. There is a line drawn on the floor between them. Each child has a collar made from a towel or piece of strong cloth placed around his neck. Each child grabs both ends of the other person's towel. The object is for each one to try to pull the other one across the line. The child who succeeds scores a point for his team. Each child on the team does the same. The team with the most points wins.

Suggested Use: This activity can be used to demonstrate the gravitational pull of earth and the moon, or the planets and the sun. It might be pointed out that a larger child was often stronger and was usually able to pull a smaller child across the line just as members of the solar system are pulled to the largest member, the sun.

Concept: Earth's Atmosphere — Air Has Pressure and Pushes Against Things

Activity: Balloon Throw

Children take turns throwing an inflated toy balloon. A line is marked on the floor, and the thrower may use any method of throwing as long as he does not step on or over this line. His throw is measured from the line to the spot his balloon first touches the floor. The child with the longest throw wins.

Suggested Use: The children can experience the feeling of throwing an object so light in relation to size that the resistance of air prevents the object from traveling in an arc as expected. In substituting a playground ball, the children can note the difference in the distance it travels with the same type of throw. A tennis ball can also be used for comparison of distance traveled and action of throwing.

Concept: Earth's Atmosphere — Force or Lift of Air

Activity: Air Lift

The children are divided into teams of four to six members each. One team stands on one side of a net stretched across the center of the court. The size of the court may vary. The game is started by one child throwing a rubber ring over the net. Any opposing team member may catch the ring and throw it back. The ring may not be relayed to another child on the same team. Play continues until a point is scored. A point is made each time the ring hits the ground in the opponent's court or when any of the following fouls are committed:

1. Hitting the net with the ring.
2. Throwing the ring under the net.
3. Relaying the ring or having two teammates touch it in succession.
4. Throwing the ring out of bounds if the opposing team does not touch it.

The team scored upon puts the ring in play again. Five to fifteen points is a game, depending on the skill of the group.

Suggested Use: The ring is used to represent an airplane, and the children's attempts to toss it over the net without allowing it to fall can be compared to *lift*. In attempting to toss the ring over the net, many fouls may be committed, and it should be pointed out that this is due to both the insufficient amount of force of air, the downward pull of gravity and also poor aiming. In most cases more force or lift is needed to launch a ring or plane. When each point is made, it can be referred to as a plane successfully launched. The children might be encouraged to find out how planes are launched from aircraft carriers. They may conclude that a plane must have an enormous lift before it can rise. It can be further pointed out that the force which produces the lift to cause a plane to rise is caused by movements of air, and that this movement produces low pressures over the top of the wings, and high pressures under the bottom of the wings.

Concept: Earth's Atmosphere — Water Cycle

Activity: Water Cycle Relay

The children are divided into teams of six children each. Each child is assigned a part of the water cycle in the order of the process — that is (1) water vapor, (2) rain, (3) land, (4) stream, (5) river and (6) ocean. The teams stand in rows close enough to be able to pass a ball from one child to the next. On a signal, the first child of each team calls his part of the water cycle (water vapor), passes the ball to the second child on his team, and runs to the end of his team's line. The second child calls out his part (rain), passes the ball to the next team member, and moves back in the same manner. This procedure continues until each team has made three complete cycles. The first team to finish wins.

Suggested Use: The cycle is represented by the children moving in turn. As the children pass the ball, it should be emphasized that the various stages are represented by each child. It is important that the children note the correct order within the cycle and situate themselves in the line accordingly. The ball represents water regardless of the form it takes within the cycle. The game may be adapted by changing the rain part of the cycle to snow or sleet, and by adding brooks and bays if the children so choose.

Concept: Earth's Surface — Coastline and Mountains Cause Ocean Currents and Winds to Change Direction

Activity: Zig Zag Run

The class is divided into teams. The teams form rows behind a starting line. Four 10 pins or other objects are placed in a line four feet apart in front of each team. On a signal the first child on each team runs to the right of the first pin and to the left of the second pin, and so in a zig zag fashion, going around the last pin. He returns to place in the same manner. The second child proceeds as the first child. If a child knocks down a pin, he must set it up before he continues. The team finishing first wins.

Suggested Use: The children on the teams can represent the ocean currents and winds. The pins can represent the coastlines and mountains. It might be helpful to use children for the objects, and they could change their positions slightly each time. The children must go around the objects in order to reach their goal. If the objects were not there, the children could travel in a straight line to the goal and back. By having to go around the objects, children show how the ocean currents and winds have to change direction when they meet obstacles.

Conditions of Life

Concept: Variety of Life — Animals Live in Many Kinds of Homes

Activity: Squirrels in Trees

With the exception of one child, the children are arranged in groups of three around the activity area. Two of the children in each group face each other and hold hands, forming a hollow tree.

The third child is a squirrel and stands between the other two children. The extra child who is also a squirrel stands near the center of the activity area. If there is another extra child, there can be two squirrels. The teacher calls, "Squirrel in the tree, listen to me. Find yourself another tree!" On the word *tree,* all squirrels must run and get into different hollow trees, and the extra squirrel also tries to find a tree. There is always one extra squirrel who does not have a tree. At different points in the game, the teacher should have the children change places. The game can then be adapted for other animals such as beavers in dams, foxes or rabbits in holes, bears in caves and the like.

Suggested Use: In playing this game, children can name other animals and the kinds of homes in which they live. They can be encouraged to figure out how they could dramatize the different types of homes animals have, as the two children form the hollow tree.

Concept: Variety of Life — Animals Move About in Different Ways

Activity: Animal Relay

The children divide into several teams. The teams stand in rows behind a line about twenty feet from a goal line. The object of the relay is for each team member to move forward to the goal line and return to his place at the rear of his team, moving as quickly as he can according to the type of animal movement assigned. Relays may be varied by the children going to the goal line and back doing imitations of the following animals:

Donkey Walk — traveling on all fours imitating a donkey's kick

Crab Walk — walking on all fours, face up

Bear Walk — walking on all fours, feet going outside the hands

Rabbit Jump — child moves forward bringing his feet forward between his hands

Elephant Walk — child bends forward, hands clasped in front with elbows straight and swinging arms like the elephant's trunk

On a signal, the teams proceed with the relay using the movement indicated by the teacher. The first team finished wins.

Suggested Use: By dramatizing the various movements of animals, children are helped to learn about the differences among animals. Children can be encouraged to figure out ways of moving to represent many types of animals.

Concept: Variety of Life — Animals Escape Their Enemies in Many Ways

Activity: Snail

The children stand in a row with the teacher as the leader at the end of the line. While singing the first verse, the leader walks around in a circle and continues to walk so that the circle becomes smaller. During the singing of the second verse, the leader reverses his direction to enlarge the circle.

> Hand in hand we circle now,
> Like a snail into his shell
> Coming nearer, coming nearer,
> In we go and in we go.
> Aren't you glad this little shell
> Keeps us all and holds us well?
>
> Hand in hand we circle now,
> Like a snail just from its shell
> Going further, going further,
> Out we go and out we go.
> Aren't you glad this little shell
> Kept us all and held us well?

Suggested Use: The concept of animals needing protection from their enemies and employing various means for protection is inherent in this activity. Children might be encouraged to find out other ways animals seek protection from their natural enemies.

Concept: Variety of Life — Wind is Moving Air and Transports Some Kinds of Seeds

Activity: Flowers and Wind

The children are divided into two teams, each team having a home marked off at opposite ends of the activity area with a neutral space between. One team represents a flower, deciding among themselves which flower they shall represent — daisies, lillies, etc. They can then walk over near the home line of the opposite team. The opposing team, representing the wind, stands in a line within their home area ready to run. They guess what the flower chosen by their opponents may be. As soon as the right flower is named, the entire team must turn and run home, the wind chasing them. Any children caught by the wind before reaching home must join the wind team. The remaining flowers repeat their play, taking a different flower name each time. This continues until all of the flowers have been caught. The teams then exchange, and the flower team becomes the wind team.

Suggested Use: In this activity some of the children represent the wind and the others represent the flowers and/or seeds. As the flowers walk to the wind home, they represent the flower growing through the summer. When the wind guesses the name of the flower, this represents the end of the growth period. As the flowers begin to run, they represent the seeds, and the children chasing them represent the wind carrying the seeds along. The flowers running also represent the seeds dispersing in different directions being borne by the wind.

Concept: Interdependence of Life

Activity: Fox and Geese

Two lines are drawn on opposite ends of the activity area. One child is the fox and stands in the center of the activity area. The other children are geese and stand behind one of the end lines. When the geese are ready, the fox calls, "Run!" and the geese must then run and attempt to cross the opposite end line before the fox can catch them. The geese are not safe until they have crossed this line. The children who are tagged by the fox must help the fox tag the remaining geese the next time. The geese who have not been tagged line up at the end line and, on a signal from the fox, run back to the original starting line. When the geese have run three times, a new fox is chosen.

Suggested Use: Through this activity the children learn that animals eat other animals as a means of survival; these types of animals are called carnivorous. The children might find out about various animals that are natural enemies and substitute their names for fox and geese.

Concept: Interdependence of Life

Activity: Spider and Flies

Two goal lines are drawn at opposite ends of the activity area and a circle equal distance between the two goal lines. The children stand around the edge of the circle, facing the center. One child, the spider, sits in the center of the circle. The other children are flies. The spider sits very still while the other children, the flies, walk or skip around the circle, clapping their hands as they go. At any time the spider may suddenly jump up and chase the flies. When he does, the flies run to either goal. A fly tagged before reaching one of the goal lines becomes a spider and joins the first spider in the circle. The original spider always gives the starting signal to chase the flies, and other spiders may not leave the circle to chase the flies until he gives this signal. The last child caught becomes the next spider.

Suggested Use: The children should be encouraged to cultivate their quickness. The spider should be urged to jump up suddenly in order to surprise the flies. In this activity the children can be helped to understand the interdependence of animals for food by the dramatizing of animals hunting each other for food and the victims seeking shelter for protection.

Concept: Interdependence of Life — Some Animals Live in Social Groups in Which They Work Together to Survive

Activity: Herds and Flocks

A starting line is drawn. The children are divided into several teams, and stand one behind the other in relay formation at the starting line. A goal line is drawn thirty to forty feet in front of the starting line. Each member of the relay team is to perform a different action while going to and from the goal line. The teacher assigns the movement to each team member — that is the first child on each team is to perform one task, the second child on each team to perform another, etc. Some of the suggested actions are

Walk with stiff knees.

Place hands on hips, hold feet together and jump.

Proceed in squat position to goal, run to starting line.

Hop on one foot.

Skip to goal, sit on floor and skip to starting line.

Swing arms in circular motion while walking quickly.

Place hands on head and run.

The signal is given for the first child from each team to proceed with his assigned action. As soon as he returns to the starting line, he touches the extended right hand of the second child on his team, then goes to the end of the line. The second child goes forth performing his designated action. Play continues until one team has had all of its members complete their performances and return to their places. This team is the winner.

Suggested Use: The children can learn in playing this game that, in order to win, all the children must cooperate and perform their different actions in an acceptable manner and as quickly as they can. This can be compared with certain animal groups whose different members perform various tasks for the safety and well-being of the group. The concept can be further integrated into the game by helping children to note that just as some of the actions in the game are difficult to do, so are some of the things that have to be done in order to survive. The children might be encouraged to find out the various roles different members of animal groups perform in order to protect the members of the group from their enemies and to obtain food. They can be helped to identify which type of group member is assigned the different role — that is the strong to hunt for food, the older for lookouts, etc.

Concept: Interdependence of Life — Animals Have to Protect Themselves from One Another

Activity: Fox and Sheep

One child is selected to be the fox who stands in his den, a place marked off on one side of the activity area. The rest of the children are the sheep. They stand in the sheepfold, another area marked off on the opposite end of the activity area. The remaining part of the activity area is called the meadow. The fox leaves his den and wanders around the meadow whereupon the sheep sally forth and, approaching the fox, ask him, "Are you hungry, Mr. Fox?" If the Fox says, "No, I'm not," the sheep are safe. When the fox says, "Yes, I am!" the sheep must run for the sheepfold as the fox may then begin to chase them. The fox tags as many sheep as he can before they find shelter in the fold. Those sheep who are caught must go to the fox's den and, thereafter, assist the fox in capturing sheep. The original fox is always the first one to leave the den. He is also the one who answers the sheep's questions. The last sheep caught becomes the fox for the next game. This game can be adapted by using other animals who are natural enemies to each other as cat and mouse, hound and rabbit, or fox and geese.

Suggested Use: In this activity the children dramatize the interdependence of animals — that some animals need others for food and are natural enemies. The children can sense the fear of the chase and the need to protect oneself. The children may find out the names of the different types of shelters of the different animals.

Chemical and Physical Changes

Concept: Movement of Molecules in Solids, Liquids and Gases
Activity: Molecule Ball

The children arrange themselves in a circle. The group then counts off by twos. The number 1's face inward, and the number 2's face outward — that is, 1's and 2's are facing each other. Each captain has a ball that is to be moved around the circle until it travels back to the captain. The exact manner in which the balls are to be moved around the circles is determined by the leader calling "solid, liquid or gas." When gas is called, the ball is to be thrown from one child to the next; when liquid is called, the ball is to be bounced from one child to the next; and when solid is called, the ball is to be passed to the next child. When the ball completes the circle, that team which does so first is declared the winner. Whenever a child drops or does not catch the ball passed to him, he must retrieve the ball, return to his place in the circle, then continue to move the ball to the next child.

Suggested Use: The use of solid, liquid and gas as call words to change the speed of the balls' progress around the circles emphasizes the difference in speed of molecules' movement in solids, liquids and gases. The children can be helped to note that the method of moving the ball around the circle relates to the speed of the movement of molecules in these different states of matter.

Concept: Molecules are in Rapid and Ceaseless Motion
Activity: Molecule Pass

The class is divided into four groups with each group standing in a straight line. The four groups form a rectangle with each group representing one side of the rectangle. The captain of each group stands near the center of the rectangle in front of his group. On a signal, each captain throws his ball to his group, starting at the right. As each child receives the ball, he throws it back to his captain and assumes a squatting position. When the captain throws the ball to the last child in his group, he runs to the right of his group as the rest of the children stand. The last child on the left runs with the ball to the captain's place, and the procedure is repeated.

Suggested Use: Each ball represents a molecule of matter. The balls are kept in motion at all times. The children can be helped to note that the ball (the molecule or matter) has to be kept moving. This can lead to a discussion of molecules of different substances, the greater space and rapid movement of molecules of gases (depending on area and temperature), the less space and less rapid movement of molecules of liquids, and the lesser space and least rapid movement of molecules of solids.

Concept: Elements in a Compound (The Composition of Molecules) Cannot Be Separated by Physical Means

Activity: Boiling Water

Two or more circles are formed. Each circle is given one or more balls. A container such as a wastebasket is set along the sidelines of the activity area. One child in each circle is the leader. When the teacher calls, "Cold water!" the children in each circle pass the ball from one child to the next. Whenever the teacher calls "Warm water!" the children roll the ball across the center of the circle from one to another. If the teacher calls, "Boiling water!" the children throw the ball to different ones in the circle. When the teacher calls "Water vapor!" the ball is immediately thrown to the circle leader who runs with it to the container on the sidelines. The team whose leader reaches the container first wins.

Suggested Use: The ball represents a molecule of water. The ball is one of the surface molecules. At first the molecule moves slowly (cold water). When the water begins to warm up, the speed of the molecule increases (warm water). As the water approaches boiling point, the speed of molecules increases (boiling water) until it acquires sufficient motion to escape to the air (water vapor). The ball (molecule) has not been altered. It has moved from one place (the liquid state or water) to another place (gaseous state or water vapor).

Concept: Chain Reaction Comes from One Molecule Hitting Another (or Neutrons in Radioactive Materials)

Activity: Tag and Stoop

The children are scattered over the activity area. One child is *it* and tries to tag two children, one with each hand. When *it* tags the first child, he then grasps the hand of that child. The two continue running after other children until *it* is able to tag a second child. *It* then stands still and gets down in a stooping position. The two children tagged now try to tag two others each, then they stoop down. The four children tagged now continue in the same manner. The object of the game is to see how long it takes for everyone to be tagged.

Suggested Use: In trying to demonstrate chain reaction, the increasingly powerful effect of a small beginning should be brought out. As the children watch the spread of those who are being tagged, they can see this effect.

Concept: Burning is Oxidation: The Chemical Union of a Fuel with Oxygen

Activity: Oxygen and Fuel

One child is chosen to be fuel and another child is oxygen. The remaining children join hands and form a circle with fuel in the center of the circle and oxygen on the outside of the circle. The children in the circle try to keep oxygen from getting into the circle and catching fuel. If oxygen gets in the circle, the children in the circle then let fuel out of the circle and try to keep oxygen in, but they must keep their hands joined at all times. When oxygen catches fuel, the game is over, and they join the circle while two other children become fuel and oxygen. If fuel is not caught in a specified period of time, a new oxygen can be selected.

Suggested Use: One child represents the fuel (as trees in a forest), and another, the oxygen (the air). The children in the circle are the preventers of fire. If oxygen catches fuel and ignites him by tagging him, a fire is started. Then the game is over. In this manner the children can be helped to note that oxygen feeds fire and that oxygen must be kept from fires that have been started in order to put them out. The children might be encouraged to find out ways that fires are smothered depending upon the type of burning material.

Light

Concept: When Light Strikes a Solid Object, It Bounces
Activity: Light Bounce

The children are divided into several teams. Two lines are marked on the activity area parallel to a blank wall. One line is drawn six inches from the wall and is the goal line. The second line is drawn twelve feet from the wall. Behind this second line, the teams stand in rows. Each team is given a small wooden block. The first child on each team takes turns throwing his block. If the block lands between the goal line and the wall, a point is scored for that team. If the block falls outside the goal line, each other team gets a point. Each child on the team proceeds in the same manner until each child has had a throw. The team with the highest score wins.

Suggested Use: Children can be helped to note that the wooden blocks rebound from the wall just as light rays do upon coming in contact with a solid object.

Concept: Heat and Light Can be Reflected
Activity: Heat and Light

The children are divided into several teams. The teams make rows at a specified distance from the blank wall of a room or the building. The first child on each team throws a ball against the wall and catches it as it bounces back to him, passes it over his head to the next child on the team, and then moves to the end of the line. The team to complete the procedure first wins.

Suggested Use: Attention can be called to the fact that light and heat are reflected just as the ball hits the wall and bounces back; light and heat are reflected or bounced off by a mirror or other shiny surface.

Concept: A Prism Can Separate a Beam of White Light Into a Spectrum
Activity: Spectrum Relay

The class is divided into two teams so that there will be seven children on each team. Each team forms a row behind a starting line. The children on each team are then assigned a specific color of the spectrum and stand in the correct order that colors appear in the spectrum — red, orange, yellow, green, blue, indigo and violet. Each child is given the appropriate color tag to pin on his clothing so that his teammates can quickly see where to line up. Those children who are not assigned to a relay team are the prism and stand at a given distance away from the starting line; they space themselves several feet apart, facing the relay teams. On a signal, all the children on each team must run between and around back of the children standing a distance away (the prism) and return to the starting line. The team must then join hands so that each team finishes by being lined up in the correct order of colors in the spectrum behind the starting line. The first team lined up correctly behind the starting line wins. A few children may change places with those who did not have a chance to run in the first relay.

Suggested Use: This relay provides children the opportunity to dramatize the concept of the prism. The teams represent the beams of light before passing through the glass prism, (represented by the children standing a distance away) and that after they passed through the glass prism, they then represented the band of colors called the *visible spectrum.* During the discussion it can be pointed out that each color of light travels through the glass prism at a different speed. The children can be encouraged to find out about different things in nature that serve as prisms to create visible spectrums.

Energy

Concept: A Body Left to Itself, Free from the Action of Other Bodies, Will, if at Rest, Remain at Rest
Activity: Pin Guard

The children form a circle. Ten pins or other suitable objects are set up in the middle of the circle. One child is selected as a guard to protect the pins. On a signal, the children start rolling a ball to knock over the pins. The guard tries to keep the ball away from the pins by kicking it back toward the circle. The child who succeeds in knocking down a pin becomes the new guard.

Suggested Use: The pins in this game represent the body at rest (inertia), and the ball, the force that puts the body in motion. It can be pointed out to the children that the pins in the center of the circle remain at rest until an outside force (the ball) strikes the pins and puts them in motion.

Concept: Friction

Activity: Siamese Twins

The children get in pairs and sit back to back with arms folded and legs extended straight ahead and together. The object is to see which pair can stand first with feet together while maintaining the folded arm position.

Suggested Use: Before the activity the children can talk about some of the results of friction such as heat and the resulting problems confronting scientists who design space missiles. The class might discuss ways in which friction helps them — that is the friction between feet and ground when one walks and how the use of snow tires or chains provides friction in snow and icy weather. During and after this activity, the teacher can help the children to see how the friction of their feet against the floor keeps them from sliding down. After the activity the children might plan to chart lists of ways in which friction helps them.

Concept: Machines Make Work Easier — Arm as Lever

Activity: Hot Potato

The class is divided into even number lines of five to six children each, separated by arm lengths from each other. Each line faces another line five to twenty feet away. Each child has a turn holding a ball at chest height in one hand and hitting it with the palm of the other hand directing the ball to the line facing him. Each child of the opposite line scores one point for each ball he catches. The child who catches the ball then proceeds to hit the ball back to the opposite line who tries to catch the ball to score a point. The child with the highest score wins.

Suggested Use: The use of the arm as a level can be demonstrated in this activity. The teacher might draw a picture on the chalkboard to show children how the arm works as a lever.

Concept: The Lever (In the Third-Class Lever the Effort is Placed Between the Load and the Fulcrum)

Concept: The Greater a Force Applied to a Mass, the Greater the Acceleration of That Mass Will Be

Activity: Net Ball (Note: Two Concepts Can Be Developed by Net Ball)

Before this activity the children can be told that serving is a basic skill used in the game of net ball, and for a successful game of net ball it is necessary to learn to serve the ball properly. The server stands on the end line facing the net. He holds the ball in his left hand about waist high in front of him and to the right. He hits the ball underhand with his right hand (heel or fist). The weight of the body is transferred forward to the left foot as the right arm moves forward in a follow-through movement. For left-handed children the procedure is reversed.

The children are divided into two groups, each group spaced in a pattern on one side of the net facing the other group. After the teacher demonstrates several times, each child is given the opportunity to attempt to serve the ball two or three times. Following practice, the game is started by one child serving the ball over the net. Any opposing team member may hit the ball with his hands back to the other side of the net. The ball may not be relayed to another child on the same team. Play continues until a point is scored. A point is scored each time the ball hits the surface area in the opponents' court or any of the following violations are committed:

1. Hitting the net with the ball
2. Hitting the ball under the net
3. Relaying the ball or having two teammates touch it in succession
4. Hitting the ball out of bounds if opposing team does not touch it

Suggested Use: (The Lever) During the practice it can be shown how the arm has acted as a lever in the serving action, that the elbow joint was the fulcrum, the forearm was the effort, and the ball was the load. Children can then be encouraged to find other examples that would illustrate this type of lever — a man swinging a golf club or a boy swinging at a ball with a bat.

Suggested Use: (Force and Acceleration) It can be noted that the servers have difficulty getting the ball in the opposite court, that the ball either fails to go over the net or it is hit out of bounds on the opposite side. The teacher can stop the activity to ask what makes the ball go out of bounds. The children might note that it was hit too hard. If the ball fails to go over the net, it can be pointed out that it was not hit hard enough. The teacher can then ask the class to explain what factor influences the speed and distance the ball travels. The force of the serve or how hard the ball is hit governs the acceleration of the ball. The children can be encouraged to apply this concept to other types of activities such as batting a baseball, peddling a bicycle or a rocket booster.

Concept: Electricity is the Flow of Electrons in a Closed Circuit
Activity: Electric Ball

The children form a circle and join hands (representing a closed circuit). The children are to move a soccer ball or similar-type ball around the inside of the circle. The ball represents the current or flow of electrons. The children move the ball from one child to the next by using the instep of the foot as in soccer. The object of the game is to keep the ball moving around the circle and preventing the ball from leaving the circle by blocking it with the feet or legs while keeping the hands joined at all times. If the ball leaves the circle (an open or broken circuit), the two children between whom the ball escapes the circle are each given a point. The game continues with the children having the lowest scores as winners.

Suggested Use: Children are able to see this concept demonstrated in this activity, that of the flow of electrons through a closed circuit by passing the ball around the circle and that a broken circuit prevents the flow of electricity when the ball leaves the circle.

Concept: Electricity is the Flow of Electrons in a Closed Circuit
Activity: Current Relay

Children are arranged in teams in rows. Each child reaches back between his legs with his right hand and grasps the left hand of the child immediately in back of him. On a signal, the teams thus joined together race to the goal line some thirty to forty feet from the starting line, then race back to the starting line. The team finishing first with the line unbroken wins.

Suggested Use: The joined hands of the members of the teams represent the closed circuit. As long as the circuit remains unbroken, electricity can flow. (The children can move their feet and procced with the race.) If the circuit is broken, it has to be repaired (the children rejoin hands) before electricity can continue to flow and the team can move forward again.

Concept: Lightning Is Electricity

Activity: Lightning Relay

The class is divided into several teams. The first child in each team toes a starting line. On a signal, he jumps. Someone marks the heel print of each jumper. The next child on each team steps forward to the heel mark of the first child, toes this mark, and jumps. This procedure is continued until every child on each team has jumped. The team having jumped the greatest distance wins.

Suggested Use: Each child is electricity or lightning *jumping* from one cloud to another. The concept of lightning being electricity gathering in a cloud and jumping to the ground or to another cloud can be noted by the children as they dramatize it in this activity.

Concept: Electricity Flows Along Metal Conductors and Will Not Flow Along Nonmetal Conductors as Glass or Rubber

Activity: Keep Away

If there is a large number of children, they should form a circle. For a small group, the children may spread out and form a square or five-sided figure. One child is chosen to be *it,* and he stands in the center. The other children throw a ball around the circle or across the square. They try to keep the ball away from *it* while he tries to get his hands on it. If *it* catches the ball he changes places with the last child who threw it, and the game continues. If *it* is unable to get hold of the ball in one minute another *it* can be chosen.

Suggested Use: The ball becomes the electricity, the ball throwers are the conductors, and *it* is a nonconductor who tries to interfere with the flow of electricity. Any time the nonconductor is successful in interfering, the current of electricity is interrupted. Children can be encouraged to find out the kind of materials that are nonconductors and several safety practices that have developed for those working around electricity, both in business and around the home.

Concept: A Magnet Attracts Iron and Steel

Activity: Link Tag

The children are scattered about the activity area. Two children are chosen to be the taggers. The taggers link hands and attempt to tag other children. All children tagged link hands between the first two taggers, the chain growing longer with each addition. Only the end children, the original taggers, may tag other children. Runners may crawl under the chain to escape being tagged, but any child who deliberately breaks the chain is automatically caught. The game continues until all the children are tagged. The last two children caught become taggers for the next game.

Suggested Use: The taggers are the magnets, and the other children represent things made of iron or steel. As the taggers touch the other children by tagging, the children are attracted to them and become a part of the magnetic chain. It should also be pointed out that only the taggers at the ends of the chain can tag others; this demonstrates that magnets are strongest at the ends or poles.

Concept: The Force of a Magnet Will Pass Through Many Materials

Activity: Hook-On Tag

One child is selected as a runner or magnet. The remaining children form groups of four. The children in each group stand one behind the other, each with arms around the waist of the child in front. The runner attempts to hook on at the end of any group of four where he can. The group members twist and swing about, trying to protect their end from being caught. If the runner is successful, the leader of that group becomes the new runner. The group having the most of its original members in it at the end of a specified period of time is the winner.

Suggested Use: Before starting the game, it should be pointed out that the runner in the game is the magnet. When he is successful in hooking onto the end of one of the groups, the power of the magnet travels through the group to the first person, and he becomes the new magnet. This activity dramatizes that a magnet does not have to be in direct contact with another magnetic material in order to attract it. Later, children can be encouraged to experiment to determine which materials the force of a magnet will travel through.

Concept: Unlike Poles of a Magnet Attract Each Other

Activity: North and South

The class is divided into two equal groups. The two groups line up facing each other about ten feet apart midway between designated goal lines. One group is named north, and the other one, south. The teacher has a ten-inch square of cardboard which has an N on one side and an S on the other. The teacher throws the cardboard into the air between the teams where all can see it as it lands. If the S side shows, the south team turns and runs to their goal line, chased by the north team. All who are tagged before reaching the line join north, and the two groups line up facing each other again. The cardboard is thrown into the air again, and the game continues in the same manner. The team which eliminates the other wins.

Suggested Use: The two groups represent the opposite or unlike poles of a magnet, the N and S poles. When one group turns to run to its goal line, it attracts the other group which pursues it.

Concept: When a Magnet Attracts an Object, That Object Becomes a Magnet

Activity: Magnet, Magnet

The children are divided into groups called pins, needles, paper clips, or anything else that can be attracted by a magnet. The groups stand behind a line at one end of the activity area. One child is selected to be the magnet and stands in the center of the activity area. The magnet calls, "magnet, magnet, I dare pins to come over" (or any of the other groups). All the children of that group run to the opposite side of the activity area. Magnet tries to catch them. Any child tagged must then help magnet whenever he calls another group to come over. The magnet may dare everybody over at one time or two groups at a time. The last child caught becomes the new magnet.

Suggested Use: The children should note that the magnet, as he tags other children, causes them to become *magnetized* and have the power to magnetize others by tagging them. The magnet *attracts* others by calling to them.

Concept: Sound Carries Through the Air

Activity: Stoop Tag

The children form a circle by joining hands. One child is *it* and stands in the center of the circle. The children walk around the circle singing,

> I am happy! I am free!
>
> I am down! You can't catch me!

At the word *down* the children stoop and let go of hands. Then they stand up and jump and hop about, daring the child who is *it* to tag them. They must stoop to avoid being tagged. If a child is tagged when he is not stooping, he becomes *it*.

Suggested Use: After the children have played the game, the teacher can discuss the sounds they have heard — singing, shouts, squeals. The teacher can question the children as to how these sounds got to them. It can be pointed out that the sounds were sound waves traveling through the air.

CHAPTER EIGHT

LEARNING IN SOCIAL STUDIES
THROUGH MOTOR ACTIVITY

THROUGHOUT the years the objectives of education have changed with the needs of society. Perhaps these changes in the objectives have had a more marked influence upon social studies than any of the other curriculum areas. In modern times one hears such statements as "education for living," "education for life in a democracy," or "education for adjustment to an ever changing world." All of these statements imply that it should be a fundamental purpose of our modern educational system to assist the child in coping satisfactorily with situations that are concerned with social relations. It is doubtful that this goal can be attained solely on the basis of having the child master a variety of geographical and historical facts. On the other hand, if the child is to function satisfactorily in social situations, it would appear to be more feasible to develop a social studies program that will provide learning experiences involving an understanding and appreciation of the social customs, mores and spiritual values as well as the interdependence of past and present peoples.

This is a large order indeed, and it is questionable whether the social studies area should be expected to cope with it alone. Certainly other curriculum areas should assume a fair share of the responsibility in the development of these understandings and appreciations.

SOCIAL STUDIES EXPERIENCES
THROUGH MOTOR ACTIVITY

Some of the objectives of the social studies program in the elementary school include (1) to help children live by democratic processes, (2) to help children learn the procedures involved in problem-solving, (3) to help children develop appreciation of

161

leadership and followership, and (4) to help children gain an understanding and appreciation of the customs and contributions of our own people as well as the people of other lands. Potential opportunities for acquiring these knowledges and appreciations are abundant in many phases of motor activity experiences. The following list suggests a number of general ways in which it is possible to utilize motor activities in social studies experiences.

1. There are numerous situations in motor activities through which children may gain a better understanding of the importance of cooperation. By their very nature many active games depend upon the cooperation of group members in achieving a common goal. Dancing is an activity that requires persons to perform together in a synchronization of rhythmical patterns. In skills such as throwing and catching there must be a coordinated action of the thrower and catcher. In certain kinds of stunts children work and learn together in groups of three, two children assisting the performer and the other taking turns in performing. In these and countless other situations, the importance of working together for the benefit of the individual and the group is readily discerned.

2. It has been demonstrated on numerous occasions that children can gain an insight into the way of life of our own people and people of other lands by learning dances, stunts and games engaged in by these people. Since active play is perhaps the one best medium for child understanding, this procedure is a particularly noteworthy one. Early American country dances and nationality dances as well as various kinds of period games and games from foreign lands provide children with an opportunity to see the significance between the activities and the cultural and physical aspects that bear upon them.

3. Group consciousness and friendliness within a group can be developed in certain motor activities. The natural opportunities for wholesome group experiences in games provide a means for the development of ability to get along with various kinds of people.

4. Certain activities help provide an understanding of the meaning and need for boundaries and zones. Games that require a

certain sized playing space where players stay in certain zones are helpful in interpreting the purpose of boundaries of countries, zoning in communities and the like.

5. Many motor activities provide an opportunity for planning and working together. Children are able to learn techniques of planning and working together when the teacher works with them in organizing and carrying out ideas for the play activities.

6. Issues that might come up as a result of certain misunderstandings in active play situations give rise to the exercise of wholesome social controls. The relationship of these social controls in play experiences to those in community living might possibly be understood in varying degrees by children at the different age levels. In these situations outstanding settings are provided for the development of problem-solving techniques in which children are placed in a position to make value judgments.

THE USE OF MOTOR ACTIVITIES IN
SOCIAL STUDIES UNITS

When the history of education is considered over a period of several hundred years, the *unit* may be thought of as a more or less recent innovation. Because of this it is difficult to devise a universal definition for the term *unit*. This is due partly to the fact that the term does not at the present time have a fixed meaning in the field of education. Essentially, the purpose of unitary teaching is to provide for a union of component related parts which evolve into a systematic totality. In other words, the unit should consist of a number of interrelated learnings which are concerned with a specific topic or central theme. A variety of types of experiences as well as various curriculum areas are drawn upon for the purpose of enriching the learning medium for all children so that the understandings of the topic in question can be developed.

There is universal agreement among educators that the things children do (the activities) are by far the most important part of the unit. Yet, those experiences through which children may actually learn best, that is, active play experiences, have been grossly neglected as essential and important activities of the unit.

It is not implied that the recommendation of the use of motor activities as learning activities of social studies is something new. In fact, a good many years ago, Mossman developed a list of things that people do.[1] These activities were classified into ten groups, with a total of some eighty different activities. It is interesting to note that some of the activities were concerned with exactly the things that children do in the form of motor activities such as *playing* and *dancing*.

In order to show more clearly how motor activities can be used as a means of extending the basis for learning in social studies units, an example is submitted at this point. This example concerns the broad areas of *periods of exploration, colonization* and *western expansion* in the development of this country. Following is a sampling of the concepts of the units and the motor activities used in the development of them.

Concept: Many people decided to settle in the western part of the country when lands were opened for homesteading; there were often exciting races for the choice sites. This concept was further developed by a game called Circle Run. In this game the players form a circle and stand about six feet apart. All face counterclockwise. On a signal all start to run, keeping the general outline of the circle. As they run, each player tries to pass the runner in front of him on the outside. A player passing another tags the one passed, and the one passed is out of the race. The last person left in the circle wins. On a designated signal from the teacher the circle turns around and runs in a clockwise direction. This may occur at the discretion of the teacher.

Concept: Many pioneers became famous for their deeds of courage and heroism. This concept was further developed through a game called Famous Pioneers. One player is selected as *it* and he has a paper pinned on the back of his clothing upon which is written the name of a famous pioneer. All of the other players stand on a line facing *it*, who

---

[1]Lois C. Mossman, *The Activity Concept.* New York, The Macmillan Company, 1938, p. 54.

has turned around so that the other players can see his pioneer name. *It* asks questions of the players until he can identify his pioneer name by their answers. When *it* guesses the name, all players run to a line at the opposite end of the activity area. *It* tries to tag as many as he can before they get across the line. Players take turns being *it*, and different pioneer names are used.

Concept: The colonists and pioneers needed great endurance and stamina to survive in the wilderness that was their new home. This concept was further developed by a combative stunt called Back-to-Back Pull. In this activity two children of nearly equal size and strength stand back to back, holding a stick with both hands over their heads. Each tries to pull the stick forward and across his own chest. A great deal of strength and endurance are often required for success. (A part of an old mop handle or broom handle can be used as the stick for this combative activity.)

Concept: Many of the skills and knowledges of the Indians were adopted by the white settlers (Indian scout pacing). This concept was further developed by the Scout Pace Relay. The class is divided into a number of equal groups, and each group forms a column. On a signal, the first person in each column travels to a given point and returns by alternating running and walking. He first runs ten paces, then walks ten paces, alternating this procedure until he returns to the original starting point. Each succeeding person in each column carries out this same procedure. The column finishing first wins.

MOTOR ACTIVITIES AS ESSENTIAL ASPECTS OF SOCIAL STUDIES UNITS

The previous discussion and examples purported to indicate how motor activities might serve to provide activities to help in developing the understandings of a social studies unit. This section of the chapter pertains to those situations in which motor activities might well be considered essentially responsible for the success of certain units. To illustrate this point, some practical examples follow. The first example pertains to a motor activity which was an outgrowth of a fifth grade social studies unit called "Living in Colonial Maryland." During one phase of this study, the pupils were divided into groups to explore the subject "Living, Working, and Playing in Colonial Days."

One group had as its problem "Good Times in Early Maryland." It was the job of this group to locate, read and study any information on this subject, and to share it with the class in any way they felt effective.

After three days of research and discussion, the children listed many colonial activities such as square dancing, handicap races and husking bees. They discovered that many of the good times in colonial days were based upon work. They read that husking bees were a very popular example, and that while the adults were husking corn, the children played games with the ears. The group members made up games and relays that the colonial boys and girls might have played at a husking bee. One of these was the Corn Race.

They decided to share their information with the other class members by having a colonial party where they taught the games enjoyed by colonial children. The food group joined them and served colonial refreshments at their party — popcorn and milk. The activity that the class preferred and requested many times afterward was the Corn Race.

In the Corn Race (a relay) the class is divided into a number of equal groups, and each group forms a column. In front of each column a circle about three feet in diameter is drawn on the activity area to represent a corn basket. Straight ahead, beyond each of the corn baskets, four smaller circles are drawn about ten feet apart. In each of the four small circles an object representing an ear of corn is placed. These objects may be blocks, beanbags or the like. At a signal, the first person in each column runs to the small circles in front of, and in line with, his column and picks up the corn one ear at a time and puts all of the ears in the corn basket. The second person takes the ears of corn from the basket and replaces them in the small circles. The third person picks them up and puts them in the basket; the game proceeds until all members have run and returned to their places.

Another example shows how folk dances were used with a third grade group as a basis for an understanding of people of other lands. The class was using a basal reader which took the children on a tour through six countries. As an introduction to the book the pupils were given a preview of the countries through travel posters and pictures. Each country was located on the map in an effort to give the children a beginning concept of life in countries beyond the boundaries of their own nation.

As study progressed and the countries were visited, many ideas were elicited from the children for learning more about the background and culture of these countries. This was done during the enrichment period of each reading lesson. A map of the world was used to advantage. As each country was visited, a small flag of that country was presented and placed on the map; a small figure of a child in the native costume was added.

One of the most enjoyable of these enrichment activities from the children's point of view was learning folk dances peculiar to the country being studied. The repertory of dances grew to such an extent that, as part of the culminating activity of the year's work, the children decided to have a folk dance festival at which time they engaged in all of the folk dances previously learned. As a further outcome, since many of these dances were those required at the annual countywide folk dance festival, learning them was placed in a much more meaningful situation.

MOTOR ACTIVITIES INVOLVING
SOCIAL STUDIES CONCEPTS

Social studies concepts are inherent in many motor activities. Inasmuch as the social studies involve topics or themes that are often closely related to the immediate environment and interests of children, there is a natural setting for integration of this curriculum area with motor activities. It has been demonstrated in numerous cases that a better understanding of concepts in certain social studies topics can be attained through participation in motor activities. The selected motor activities that appear on the following pages have been used successfully in practical situations for this purpose.

The following is a summary of activities which contain social studies concepts. Descriptions of the activities follow the summary.

Activity	Topic	Concept
Air Raid	Communication	People communicate by telephone, newspaper, radio, television, mail, etc.; the radio brings us news.
Automobile	Transportation	Man travels by automobile.
Dog Chase	Pets	Some dogs make good pets.
Meet at the Switch	Transportation	Understanding trains, tracks, and switches.
Railroad Train	Transportation	Man travels by train.
Airplanes	Transportation	Man can travel in the air by airplane.
Creative Movements	Transportation	We have many methods of transporting people and goods such as airplanes, trains and boats.
Leaves of Green	Fall	The different seasons of the year bring about changes in nature.
Row, Row, Row Your Boat	Transportation	Man can travel by water.
Newboy and Postman	Communication	The newsboy and postman deliver news to us.
Explorer	Geography	Understanding that there are seven continents.
Scouts and Indians	Colonial Life	The pioneers were sturdy people; sometimes they had to fight unfriendly Indians.
Streets and Alleys	Transportation	Our community has roadways for travel.
Community Relay	Protection	Our ways of living come through responsibility of community living by aid of security and protection.
Merry-Go-Round	Interdependence for achievement	To accomplish certain things people should work together.
Once and Over	Geography	Mountains presented a natural obstacle to the pioneers.
Stick Wrestle	Geography	Each country has a definite boundary.

Concept: People communicate by telephone, newspaper, radio, television, etc.; the radio brings us news.
Activity: Air Raid

The players form a double circle, all facing the center. One child acts as the radio voice. He is *it,* and he takes his place in the center of the circle. When *it* calls out, "Air raid!" the inside circle walks, skips or runs clockwise within the circle. When *it* calls, "All clear!" each player immediately stops in front of another player in the outside circle. *It* attempts to find a partner and the player left without a partner selects the player to be the radio voice for the next time. Each time the game is played, the inside and outside circles are alternated.

Concept: Man travels by automobile.

Activity: Automobile

The players sit on chairs arranged in a circle. Each child is given the name of a part of an automobile such as the wheel, hub, axle and the like. The teacher or a pupil begins the game by telling a story about the automobile, bringing in the parts of it. As each part is mentioned, the child or children involved get up and run around the chair. At some point in the story, the storyteller calls out, "Automobile!" At this point everyone must leave his seat and get a different one, with the storyteller trying to get to one of the seats. The person who does not get a seat can become the storyteller, or a point can be scored against him, as the children decide.

Concept: Some dogs make good pets.

Activity: Dog Chase

The class is divided into five or six groups. The members of each group are given the name of a dog such as collie, poodle and the like. The small groups then mingle into one large group. One child acting as the leader throws a ball or other object away from the groups, at the same time calling out one of the dog names. All of the children with this dog name run after the thrown object. The one who gets possession of it first becomes the leader for the next time.

Concept: Understanding trains, tracks and switches.

Activity: Meet at the Switch

One child selected as the trainmaster stands in front of the group with an object such as a ball, beanbag or the like in each hand. The other players form into two teams in columns, with the first player on each team on the starting line. When the leader gives a signal, the first two players of each team run up and each takes an object out of the leader's hand. They turn and run in opposite directions around the two columns, meeting at the back of the columns as trains at a switch. They stop and shake hands or perform some other activity in which both are involved, then proceed in the same direction they were going. The player who replaces the object in the hand of the leader first is the winner and scores a point for his team. The game proceeds until all of the players have had a turn. The scores of each team are then totaled and the team with the highest score is the winner.

Concept: Man travels by train.

Activity: Railroad Train

One child is selected to be the trainmaster and another to be the starter. The rest of the children are given the names of parts of a train, workers, kinds of trains or objects carried on a train. The trainmaster then tells a story using the names that have been given to the children. When a child's train name is mentioned, he runs to the starter and stands behind him, putting his hands on the shoulders or hips of the child in front of him. When all have become a part of the train, or whenever the starter wishes, he gives the starting whistle and the train starts moving around the activity area. The starter leads the train wherever he wishes it to go.

Concept: Man can travel in the air by airplane.

Activity: Airplanes

The group is dispersed around the activity area, each child taking a squatting position with the arms out to the side. To the accompaniment of a drum or a recording the children walk in the squat position, and as the accompaniment speeds up and becomes louder they rise to a standing position as if airborn.

Concept: We have many methods of transporting people and goods such as airplanes, trains and boats.

Activity: Creative Movements

Various kinds of transportation motivate creative movement expression. Airplanes, boats, trains and the like have numerous possibilities of movements that children enjoy. The activities of these various means of transportation can be worked out in movement, much of which can be creative on the part of the children.

Concept: The different seasons of the year bring about changes in nature.

Activity: Leaves of Green

The children join hands and form a circle. They walk around the circle counterclockwise while singing the following verse to the tune of "Here We Go Round the Mulberry Bush,"

> We have leaves of green and nuts of brown
> That hang up high but will not come down.
> If we leave them alone until fall weather,
> Why then they will all come down together.

After the last word *together* is sung, the children all shout, "Whoops!" and drop to a stooping position in the manner of falling nuts.

Concept: Man can travel by water.

Activity: Row, Row, Row Your Boat

The children stand in four rows and place their hands on the shoulders of the child in front of them. The children in each row sing one or more rounds of the song. The following action is carried out as each row begins its first round of singing.

1. Row, row, row your boat,
   (The first row of children takes four steps forward in unison.)
2. Gently down the steam.
   (The second row of children takes four steps forward and the first row takes four steps backward to its original place.)
3. Merrily, merrily, merrily,
   (The third row of children takes four steps forward, the second row takes four steps backward, and the first row takes four steps forward.)
4. Life is but a dream.
   (The fourth row of children take four steps forward, the third row takes four steps backward, the second row takes four steps forward, and the first row takes four steps backward.)

This procedure is continued until all of the rounds have been sung. All rows will then be back in their original positions.

Concept: The newsboy and postman deliver news to us.

Activity: Newsboy and Postman

This activity involves such fundamental skills as walking, running and skipping. Some of the children impersonate a newsboy and some a postman. They do this by doing many things a newsboy does such as piling up papers, throwing folded papers on stoops and porches, and the like. In impersonating the postman they do such things as lifting the mailbag on their shoulders, lifting packages and the like. They also walk, run and skip as a newsboy might in delivering his papers.

Concept: Understanding that there are seven continents.

Activity: Explorer

The players are seated in a circle with one player in the center of the circle. Each player selects the name of one of the continents and tells its name. (Several children will have the name of the same continent.) The explorer, standing in the center of the circle, calls out the name of two continents. The children who have these names must get up and get a different seat. The explorer tries to get a seat, and the player left without a seat selects the explorer for the next time.

Concept: The pioneers were sturdy people; sometimes they had to fight unfriendly Indians.

Activity: Scouts and Indians

The class is divided into two teams. Two lines are drawn parallel about twenty-five to thirty feet apart with each team standing behind each of the lines. The area between the two lines is the neutral area. One team is called the scouts, and the other team is called the Indians. The scouts' territory is called the stockade, and the Indians' territory is called the Indian village. Either scouts or Indians venture into the neutral area, and when they do they run the risk of being caught by the enemy. Members of either team, either individually or in small groups, attempt to bring opponents back to their own territory. That is, the Indians try to capture the scouts and take them to the Indians village, and the scouts try to capture the Indians and take them to the stockade. The team with the greatest number of prisoners after a specified period of time is the winner. (If players fail to venture into the neutral area, the teacher should devise a signal denoting that a certain number of them should go into that area; otherwise the objective of the game is lost.)

Concept: Our community has roadways for travel.

Activity: Streets and Alleys

The children stand in several columns facing the leader who stands in front of the group. When they are standing in this position, the aisles between the columns are called streets. When the entire group turns ninety degrees to the right, the aisles between them are called alleys. In this position they join hands with the child on either side. The position of the group can be changed by the leader. That is, when he calls, "Streets!" they take a position one behind the other facing the front. When he calls "Alleys!" they turn ninety degrees to the right and stand side by side, joining hands. A runner and a chaser are selected, and to start the game the chaser stands in front of the group, and the runner stands in back of the group. At a signal, the chaser attempts to catch the runner. They both must run up and down the aisles formed by the group. The course of the chaser and runner is changed by the leader calling out either "Streets!" or "Alleys!" Chasers and runners should be changed frequently, particularly if the chaser is having a difficult time tagging the runner.

Concept: Our ways of living come through responsibility of community living by aid of security and protection.

Activity: Community Relay

The class is arranged in column formation with from five to six children in a column. The first player in each column stands toeing a starting line. Another line is designated a given distance away. The first player runs to this line, and on the way back he must impersonate some form of community protection such as a policeman, fireman or the like. This procedure is continued until all players in each column have had an opportunity to run. The team finishing first wins. If advisable, the impersonations that the players make may be designated before the race starts.

Concept: To accomplish certain things people should work together.

Activity: Merry-Go-Round

Six children lie on their backs in the form of spokes of a wheel with feet inward and touching in the middle as a hub. One child stands between each two that are in the lying position. The persons who are standing reach down and join hands with the persons who are lying on each side of them. It is recommended that the children grasp one another's wrists. The children in the lying position straighten their bodies until only the heels are in contact with the surface area. The children in the standing position walk clockwise, and the children who are in the lying position move their heels slightly to keep the merry-go-round going. After a time, the children who are standing alternate with those who are lying.

Concept: Mountains presented a natural obstacle to the pioneers.
Activity: Once and Over

This activity involves a ball-bouncing skill that may be carried on in the classroom. A wastebasket is placed behind a chair or other suitable obstacle. The child attempts to bounce an inflated rubber ball over the chair and into the basket.

Concept: Each country has a definite boundary.
Activity: Stick Wrestle

Two lines are drawn on the surface area from five to six feet apart. Two children of equal size and strength stand in between this space, each grasping a stick. (An old mop handle or broom handle is suitable for this activity or any kind of stick that is sturdy and has a smooth surface.) At a signal, each child attempts to hold on to the stick and, at the same time, attempts to pull the stick (with his opponent) over the line.

CHAPTER NINE

LEARNING ABOUT HEALTH AND
SAFETY THROUGH MOTOR ACTIVITY

THE areas of health education and safety education are no doubt broad enough in scope to be considered and discussed as separate entities in the school program. However, because of their close relationship and because so many aspects of safety are concerned with health, the two terms health and safety are often used together.

A good many years ago the World Health Organization defined *health* as a "state of complete physical, mental and social well being and not merely the absence of disease or infirmity." Various *safety* measures need to be taken in order to help school children approximate this level of well-being. Moreover, the area of safety concerns certain aspects which threaten the individual's health as well as those factors which contribute to his security for healthful living.

For several years the schools have accepted varying degrees of responsibility in health education in attempting to help children \develop to their greatest possible capacities. In more recent years it has been recognized that safety ranks in the same category of importance in the attempt to assure optimum growth and development of children. Consequently, if teachers think in terms of providing for the optimum health of children, they will assume responsibility in the area of safety education as they do in health education.

HEALTH AND SAFETY EXPERIENCES
THROUGH MOTOR ACTIVITY

It has been demonstrated many times over that pleasurable exercise is an essential need in stimulating the growth and development of children. It is pretty much common knowledge that muscles of the body grow in strength, size and endurance as a result of enjoyable physical activity. Also, this kind of activity favorably influences such vital organs of the body as the heart and lungs, thus improving the performance of the circulatory and respiratory systems. Indeed, children during periods of organized active play are engaging in activities which are designed to maintain and improve their health status.

It is important that children be made aware of the health values resulting from participation in motor activities. It should mentioned here that this idea is not of recent origin. In fact, a strong recommendation in this connection is found in the following statement made by Warnock many decades ago.

> No one, I think, would question the fact that skill in motor activities and joy in participation in those activities are important factors in healthful living. And on the other hand any motor activity program which excludes all reference to or consideration of physical, mental, social, and spiritual health, and makes no pretense at developing socially desirable attitudes, habits, and knowledges, is unworthy of the name "physical education."[1]

Teachers should not rely entirely upon the children themselves to develop an appreciation of the contribution that motor activity makes to health. On the contrary, teachers should avail themselves of every opportunity to interpret the health values of motor activity to children. If this was done in a systematic manner throughout the various educational levels, one might speculate that an appreciation for and a zeal to participate in pleasurable physical activity and exercise might be carried on into adult life.

In order to give the reader some insight into the use of motor activity in the development of health and safety concepts, some representative examples are presented here.

The first example is concerned with the health concept, *the skin is the first line of defense of the body against infectious agents.* An active game to develop the concept is Body Rebels. In the center of a large activity area a circle with a three-foot radius is

---

[1]Florence M. Warnock, Opportunities for teaching health in the elementary school through motor activities. *Journal of Health and Physical Education*, October, 1934, p. 15.

drawn. One child is chosen to be the body and stands in the center of the circle. Four children are selected to be the skin and stand outside the circle. The other children are germs and station themselves about the activity area nearer the boundary lines than the skin. The germs try to run past the skin, gain entrance to the circle and tag the body. If the body is tagged, the game ends and the child who tagged the body becomes the body for the next game. If a skin tags a germ as he tries to get into the circle to reach the body, the germ must go to the boundary line, stand still and count to 10 before he may continue to play. The skin trys to tag the germs only when they are near the circle. Once a germ enters the circle, he is safe to tag the body.

In this activity the children can dramatize that the body tries to resist invasion of bacteria into the body. The skin tries to protect the body from infection (being tagged). The germs are the infectious agents that sometimes get into the body causing illness. It can also be pointed out that as long as the skin remains intact, it wards off harmful disease agents and prevents infection from entering the body. The children can be encouraged to find out how breaks in the skin are taken care of to prevent bacteria from entering the body.

The second example shows how the game Ball Pass Relay can be used to introduce the concept, *organs are groups of tissues working together to perform major functions of the body.* Several circles are formed. The captain of each circle holds a ball. On a signal, the captain passes the ball to the right. The ball continues around the circle until it returns to the captain who immediately raises his hand. The team finishing first scores a point. Variations can be used, such as (1) passing to the left, (2) passing the ball around the circle three or four times, (3) changing the type of passes, or (4) increasing the size of the circle to make passes longer.

In applying this activity to the concept, the circles can be designated as the heart, lungs or other organs of the body. Each child can be compared to a tissue. Just as coordination and cooperation are necessary between the children in the circles in winning the game, so these same qualities are necessary for tissues in order that the organs can perform their functions. The variations in the game may suggest that just as some of the skills are more difficult to perform than others, so are some of the functions of the organs of the body more difficult to accomplish. But, with all of the tissues (and team members) working together, the difficult tasks can be accomplished.

The following tape recorded dialogues between pupils and teacher are presented to help point up the general idea more clearly. The first procedure shows how a second grade teacher used the active game, Run for Your Supper, during the course of a unit on foods.

Teacher: We sometimes hear people say that a healthy child is a hungry child. How many of you boys and girls run into the house quickly when your mother calls you to come in and eat?

Pupil: Sometimes I don't want to go in and eat because I have more fun playing.

Teacher: Yes, and I believe that is true for most children. However, we need to have strong muscles so that we can play. Because of this we need to eat certain kinds of foods, and perhaps we should eat at regular times. Now we are going outside, and I want to tell you about a new game we are going to play. The name of the game is Run for Your Supper. Why would this be a good game for us to learn just at this time?

Pupil: Because we are studying about food and how it makes you feel like playing if you eat right.

Teacher: Yes, that's right, and what does the name of this game make you think of?

Pupil: That you should hurry in to eat when you are called.

Pupil: You just said that we need strong muscles to play, so kids should take time out to eat.

Teacher: Very good, Tom. An automobile would soon quit running if we didn't put gas in it, wouldn't it? Now, I am going to explain the game to you here in the room, and I want to see if you can remember how to play it when we get outside. We will form a circle and hold hands. One person chosen to be *it* will suddenly stop between two children and say, "Run for your supper." Those two will run in different directions around the circle. They will see which one of them can get back first to the place he left. The person to get back first can select *it* for the next time.

Pupil: This game is something like another one we played. I can't remember the name.

Teacher: Does anyone remember the name of that game?

Pupil: I think it was Slap Jack.

Teacher: Yes, that was it.

Pupil: I don't see how you do this.

Pupil: Neither do I.

Teacher: Very well, let's take a little time so some of you can show how we do it. Rose, Otto and Ronny, come and stand in front of the room, please. Rose you be *it* and show us what happens.

Pupil: No, that won't work. They can't run if their hands are being held.

Pupil: How about if we put our hands on the two players' shoulders and said, Run for your supper? Everyone would know then that I was really *it*.

Teacher: I think that is a fine idea. Shall we try it that way? (The children proceed to the playground and participate in the game for a time, and then the teacher evaluates it with them.)

Teacher: Shall we review some of the things we learned in the game. Can someone tell us, Kathy?

Pupil: We make a circle, and *it* runs and chooses two to run. The next *it* is chosen by the last one back.

Teacher: Do you think the game Run for Your Supper will help you remember anything about what we are studying?

Pupil: Well, you should come in and eat when you are called instead of staying out to play some more.

Teacher: Can you give us a reason for that, Paul?

Pupil: Well, then you will be able to play more because you need food to be strong and play games.

Pupil: Good food helps make you strong, and maybe if you were hungry you would run faster.

Teacher: That might be. Can you think of ways we could make the game better?

Pupil: Try not to run into each other.

Teacher: Yes. Can you think of any way we could change this game so the players could have more turns?

Pupil: Couldn't we have more circles and have someone *it* for each one?

Teacher: That sounds like a good idea. Why don't we try that when we play a circle game again.

The second procedure illustrates how a better understanding about certain aspects of safety from poisonous plants might be developed with a game called Poison.

Teacher: Well, boys and girls, it certainly looks like spring is here with the lawns starting to get pretty and green.

Pupil: It sure does, and spring is my favorite time of year.

Pupil: Mine too. I like to walk in the woods and hunt for flowers.

Pupil: And snails and turtles, too.

Teacher: There are also some other things one might find in the woods this time of year. Do you know what they might be?

Pupil: Spiders?

Teacher: Well, yes, but I was thinking of something else that grows like plants or flowers.

Pupil: You mean moss or honeysuckle or something like that?

Teacher: Well, yes, but what I had in mind was something not quite so nice and pretty.

Pupil: Oh! Are you thinking of poison ivy?

Teacher: Right, Jack, and also poison oak and sumac. I wonder if some of you have had trouble with one of these three, or at least know someone who has.

Pupil: My brother had it, too.

Teacher: I can see that many of you know something about these three enemies of ours, and so this new game we are going to play this morning should have real meaning.

Pupil: What is the name of the game?

Teacher: It is well-named I think. It is called Poison. To play it we first join hands and form a circle. (Children form a circle.) Now, I will draw a circle on the inside of your circle about a foot in front of your toes. You will remain with your hands grasped, and on the signal, "Go!" you will try to pull someone into the circle. Anyone who steps into the circle is said to be poisoned. As soon as a person is poisoned someone calls out, "Poison!" and the one who is poisoned becomes *it* and gives chase to the rest of you. Those of you who are being chased will run to various places designated as *safety*, such as wood, stone, metal or something of that nature. All persons tagged are poisoned and become chasers. After those not tagged have reached safety, I will call out, "Change!" and they must run to another place of safety. Those poisoned attempt to tag as many as possible. We will continue the game until all but one have been poisoned. (Following a brief question-answer session to clear up some of the things about how to play the game, the teacher asks what they shall use for safety.)

Pupil: Let's use wood and metal for safety.

Teacher: All right, Fred, wood and metal it is. Now let's start the game on the signal, Go!

(The children participate in the game after which the teacher evaluates it with them.)

Teacher: Now that you have played Poison, is there anything you might think of to improve it?

Pupil: Maybe if you drew the circle a little farther away from our circle it might be tougher to be poisoned.

Teacher: Yes, you might be right, Tom; another six inches or so might help.

Pupil: I think we have too many safe places. It makes it hard for the chasers.

Teacher: Perhaps we could cut it down to one type of material. I wonder how this game will help you in relation to some of the poison plants we talked about.

Pupil: Well, for one thing, staying out of the circle is like staying on the path in the woods and not getting into the bushes.

Teacher: That's right, Frank. Even though we might not know what sumac and ivy look like, we will perhaps be much safer if we stay on the path.

Pupil: I heard that you can catch poison ivy from other people if they have it on their clothes or something like that.

Teacher: Perhaps then we should also avoid coming in contact with anyone who has been poisoned, for we might be affected that way too.

Pupil: Just like in the game; I didn't get pulled into the circle, but Jimmy did, and he touched me and I was poisoned.

Teacher: Yes, we must be careful in many ways in the summer to avoid the discomfort caused by poison ivy, poison oak and poison sumac.

These illustrations are representative of the numerous

possibilities for using motor activities in the form of active games as a learning medium in the development of health concepts.

THE USE OF MOTOR ACTIVITY IN HEALTH UNITS

There are various ways of organizing and providing health learning experiences for children. One of these procedures which has been used quite successfully in practical situations is the unit method of teaching. As mentioned in the previous chapter, the essential purpose of unitary teaching is to provide for a union of component-related parts which evolve into a systematic totality. In health education this means that the health unit will consist of a number of interrelated learnings which are concerned with a specific topic or central theme. This implies that the health unit involves a learning situation with regard to a certain area of health. Numerous types of experiences as well as various subject matter areas are used with the idea of enriching the learning situation for children so that the health concepts involved in a given topic will be more thoroughly developed.

An important feature in the construction of a health unit is the development of the framework of the unit. The framework may be referred to by various terms, some of which include *outline, sequence, guidelines* and *pattern.* Irrespective of the terms by which the framework is called, its main purpose is to include the major headings of the unit. In recent years a number of recommendations for the unit framework have been proposed and successfully used in various situations. It is recommended that teachers develop a type of unit framework which best suits their own individual needs. For purposes here the following framework developed by the author will be used because of its conduciveness to the use of motor activities.

1. Overview
2. Objectives
3. Techniques for the Discovery of Needs
4. Introduction
5. Learning Activities and Experiences
6. Evaluation
7. References (for both the teacher and pupils)

8. Materials Needed

Of the eight major headings listed above, numbers 1 through 6 are most applicable for use of motor activities, particularly in the form of active games. The discussion which follows is intended to show through examples how active games can, in certain specific ways, be an important part of each of these six headings of the unit.

Overview

It is the purpose of the overview to set forth a general statement with respect to the nature and scope of the unit. This might include a brief description of the theme of the unit as well as reasons why it is an important area of study. The following is an example of an overview of a unit entitled "Safety on Our School Playground":

> According to accident statistics, there is a great need for schools to place emphasis on various aspects of safety. Many schools are doing this, and it is perhaps one of the main reasons why in some cases the rate of accidental deaths of children in the 5 to 14-year age range is decreasing.
>
> It has been found that many school accidents occur on the playground. Because of this there is a need for certain playground regulations and understandings in order that a school may have as safe a playground as possible.
>
> In order to have a safer playground, our first grade is going to study "How to Play Safely on the Playground." It is hoped that we will be able to establish some regulations that we ourselves can use and that others in the school will want to know about and abide by.

Objectives

The objectives of the unit are the things that we want pupils to learn. In reality these things are valid health concepts that the teacher should help to develop with children. When valid health concepts are stated as objectives, they should be thought of as the teacher's goals. It is the function of the teacher to provide a classroom environment and skillful guidance in such a way that the pupils will adopt the objectives or valid health concepts as their own purposeful goals. Following is a partial list of objectives (in this case valid *safety* concepts) of the previously mentioned unit on "Safety on Our School Playground."

1. Children should wait until the bus has come to a complete stop before crossing the safety waiting line.

2. When running on the playground we should always look where we are going.

3. We should always stop, look and listen and make sure the way is clear before crossing the street.

It was found through experimentation that these concepts could be further developed through the use of active games as follows:

Concept: Children should wait until the bus has come to a complete stop before crossing the safety waiting line. This concept was further developed by the game Bus Stop. In this game twelve to fifteen children form a circle with each of these children representing a bus. Twelve or fifteen more children form an inner circle; they represent the people in the bus. One child is selected to be *it* and goes to the center of the circle; he represents an imaginary moving bus. *It* walks around fast, then slower and slower until he comes to a complete stop. When *it* stops, he represents a bus stopping; all of the children must then walk to a new bus (members of outer circle) while *it* also tries to get a bus. There will always be one player left without a bus. This player chooses the new moving bus, and the game continues.

Concept: When running on the playground, we should always look where we are going. This concept was further developed by the game Old Lady Witch. In this activity two lines are needed; one is a base line and the other line is where Old Lady Witch lives. One child is selected to be Old Lady Witch. The other players walk up to Old Lady Witch's line and ask, "What time is it, Old Lady Witch?" She answers different times, such as six o'clock, nine o'clock and so on. If she says, "twelve o'clock" or "midnight" all of the children run back to the base line. If Old Lady Witch tags any of them before they get there, they help her catch the rest of the players as the game is continued. As the children line up in front of Old Lady Witch, they should be taught how to stand in a safety line. That is, no one should stand behind other players. This is done so that when a player turns around he will be less likely to bump into another player.

Concept: We should always stop, look and listen and make sure the way is clear before crossing the street. (Sometimes a ball goes into the street and needs to be retrieved.) This concept was further developed by playing the game Red Light. In this game one child is selected to be a policeman. The other children stand on a line called the curbing. The policeman counts, "One, two, three, four, five (or more)," and turns around quickly and says either, "Red Light" or "Green Light." (He may hold up the color instead of saying the words.) As soon as the other players hear the policeman counting, they may leave the curb and keep walking until he says, "Red Light." Then they must stand very still. If the policeman sees any of the players move, he sends them back to the curb to start over. Children who are not seen moving when the policeman calls "Red Light" remain in place. The game continues and the first player to reach the curb where the policeman is standing wins the game. (Locomotor skills of hopping, jumping, running, skipping or galloping can be substituted for walking.)

Techniques for the Discovery of Needs

For the satisfactory guidance of health learning experiences of children, it is essential that teachers know their needs. For the most part, teachers are familiar with the general health needs of children. However, teachers should always be on the alert to detect specific needs as they observe children in the school environment.

Motor activity experiences can be rich in possibilities for observing children and determining some of their health needs. For example, as children engage in active games the teacher might watch for deviations from safe and healthful practices such as unsafe practices on the playground and playground equipment and whether or not children attend to matters involving cleanliness after engaging in vigorous activities. It is also possible for the competent teacher to determine the level of health knowledge of children as they engage in certain active games. In this particular connection one teacher made a critical observation of a group of first-grade children when she taught them a game called Let's Eat. In this game, the children form a close circle by standing shoulder to shoulder so that there is no open space between pupils. Each child assumes the name of a fruit or vegetable. The teacher or child selected as the leader walks around the outside of the circle calling names of fruits and vegetables. The children whose fruit and vegetable names are called follow behind the leader. When the teacher or leader calls, "Let's eat," the players attempt to get back to their original places in the circle. If the leader is successful in getting another child's place, that child selects the leader for the next time, and the game continues.

During the evaluation phase of the lesson, the teacher found that some children did not know about many of the fruits and vegetables that had been used as names in the game. In some instances, the children did not know the difference between fruits and vegetables. In this case, the active game served as a technique for the discovery of a specific need. As a result, the teacher developed a unit on foods with emphasis upon different kinds of fruits and vegetables.

Introduction

There are several ways that health units can be successfully introduced. It is extremely important that the teacher understand that the success of a unit may depend entirely upon the way it is introduced. Because of this, there are certain basic considerations that should be dealt with when deciding upon a suitable introductory activity for a particular unit topic. Insofar as possible, the introduction should be of a problem-solving nature. Also, a kind of introduction should be used in which pupils find purposeful goals.

Undoubtedly, the best approach to a unit on health is one that is derived from the immediate environment. When this is not possible, the teacher should attempt to create as suitable an environment as possible for the proper introduction.

The use of active games in the introductory phase of health

units is a practice that holds a great deal of promise. However, it is a practice that is not very prevalent at the present time. Since one of the main purposes of the introductory phase of the health unit is to arouse interest in the ensuing learning experiences of the unit, it should not be too difficult to see why active games might well be considered very valuable introductory activities. The following example is submitted to illustrate this point:

In a unit on fire protection during Fire Prevention Week, the game Forest Fire was very successfully used as an introduction to the unit. In this game, the pupils form a double circle, with all of the players facing the center. The players on the inside are the trees. Each player in the outside circle stands immediately behind a tree. One of the pupils is selected to be the lookout; he takes his position in the center of the circle. The lookout calls out, "Fire in the forest, everybody run!" He then begins to clap his hands. The players forming the outside circle behind the trees run to the left. They continue to run around the circle once, twice or three times until the lookout stops clapping. When the lookout stops clapping, he takes a place in front of one of the trees. The runners try to do the same, but one runner will be left without a tree. He selects a lookout for the next time, and the game continues with the players who were the trees becoming the runners.

After the game was played, the teacher guided the children into a discussion of fire protection. Questions by the pupils about control of fire, combating fire and the like developed into a teacher-pupil planning session and the study of fire prevention began with a high level of interest.

Learning Activities and Experiences

The things that children *do* in order to learn are considered learning activities. The personal feelings that they have from engaging in these activities are learning experiences. Needless to say, the learning activities and experiences should be considered as the most important part of the unit because it is this part that includes the major portion of things that might be learned.

One of the desirable features of the unit method of teaching in health education is that individual differences may be provided for by use of a variety of learning activities. Some of these learning activities may be peculiar to a particular subject-matter area. Strangely enough, those experiences through which many children tend to learn best — *active play experiences* — have, in many cases, been neglected as important learning activities of units.

In attempting to determine the most desirable learning activities for a given health unit, the teacher should carefully examine the objectives of the unit. It will be recalled that the objectives are valid health concepts that the teacher desires to have the children develop. Perhaps one concept might be developed best by a demonstration, and another by the use of visual aids. In many cases, it is desirable to use several learning activities to further develop a particular concept.

Game activities should be given serious consideration for their value as learning activities in further developing health concepts. The use of active games to develop the concepts in the unit on "Safety on Our School Playground" mentioned previously in this chapter is an example.

Evaluation

The evaluation phase of a health unit involves an appraisal of the learning that took place as a result of the unit. In other words, the teacher attempts to make a valid estimate of the educative growth of pupils.

The use of active games as evaluative techniques for appraisal of learning in health is an infrequent practice. Consequently, validating evidence for support of this procedure is somewhat scarce. However, some experimentation with this method has shown much promise. A couple of examples are given here for the purpose of illustrating this point. These examples might be used as points of departure for the reader to engage in further experimentation in this evaluation procedure.

One effective means of appraising health knowledge is through *dramatization*. This procedure seems to be particularly successful with children at the primary level. One aspect of dramatization that has been used with success in evaluating learning in health is the *story play.* The teacher might start a story which summarizes the learning experiences of a given health unit, and the children play or act out the story. After the story is introduced, the teacher merely guides it while the children make their own contributions to it through story-telling and story-playing. Through this evaluation procedure the teacher is able to determine to a certain extent what was learned from the unit by noting the reactions of the children.

A second example is one in which a teacher used a game called Supermarket to help appraise learning in an upper elementary unit on Food. This game is played by giving each child a food name such as milk, apple and the like. The teacher or a pupil starts the game by saying, "I am going to the supermarket to buy some food for ———." (The teacher can use any purpose for the food, such as food for breakfast, food for a picnic, food to bake a pie and the like.) When the purpose of the food is stated, the children with the food names for that purpose run to a designated area on the playground. For example, if it was food for breakfast, children with such food names as cereal, hot cakes and the like would run to the designated area. The teacher can use this procedure for knowledge about food and diet involving food selection, food classification, vitamin content, the four food groups and the like. The teacher can appraise learning by observing the reactions of the children.

SELECTED MOTOR ACTIVITIES
INVOLVING HEALTH CONCEPTS

It has been suggested throughout this chapter that there are a number of health concepts that might be developed by children as they engage in certain motor activities. Moreover, a number of examples of some of these possibilities have been given. The list that follows is a summary of additional activities along with topical areas and concepts. Descriptions of the activities follow the summary of them. In some cases specific applications for the activities are suggested. In others, just the activity and concept is given and it is suggested that the reader work out his own application for specific situations.

Activity	Topic	Concept
Germ and Toothbrush	Dental Health	One of the ways of preventing tooth decay is brushing the teeth soon after eating.
Hot Potato	Body Function	Our brain sends us messages to tell us to react quickly, protecting us from danger.
Circle Pass Ball	Disease	Cold germs are spread by direct contact. One way of preventing spread of colds is to keep away from others when you have a cold.
Change Circle Relay	Food	A balanced diet is good for health.
Ball Pass	Body Function	Circulation of the blood through the body helps the blood perform many functions.
Hook On Tag	Disease	We need to guard against disease.
Policeman	Pedestrian Safety	There are many devices used as a means of safety, one of which is the traffic light.
Dinner's Ready	Food	Children should know the importance of a proper diet.
Dog Catcher	Safety	Caution in playing with strange animals is necessary.
Get Together	Body Structure	Various parts of the body are identified by different names.
Cross the Street	Pedestrian Safety	We should always look up and down the street before crossing to make sure no cars are coming.
Fire in the House	Fire Prevention	Fire can be harmful and destructive, and we must guard against this.
Fireman	Safety Friends	Firemen put out fires.
Fruit Basket	Food	We should eat certain foods

		to grow strong and healthy.
Hill Dill	Exercise and Play-ground Safety	Outdoor play is important to good health (exercise.) Always watch where you are going in a running and tag game (playground safety.)
Attention	Body Mechanics	Erect posture is important in daily living. A strong, well-balanced framework can assume different positions. Muscles along the framework hold the body in good balance with little effort.

Concept: One of the ways of preventing tooth decay is brushing the teeth soon after eating.

Activity: Germ and Toothbrush

About ten to twelve players join hands in a semicircle. Another player stands in the middle of the semicircle, shuts his eyes and counts to ten. He then tries to find the one hiding and gives chase to him. The players in the semicircle let the chaser in and out as he chooses, but try to keep out the one being chased. The game can continue until the one chased is caught or a new chaser is named. The children who are standing in the semicircle holding hands are the teeth in the mouth. The chaser is the toothbrush. The other player, the one hiding and fleeing, is the germ. The toothbrush tries to catch the germ hiding in the mouth. The teeth help the toothbrush.

Concept: Our brain sends us messages to tell us to react quickly, protecting us from danger.

Activity: Hot Potato

All players stand in a circle. A ball or beanbag is passed rapidly from one player to another around the circle. Following it are three or four other balls or beanbags, each starting at a different place in the circle. Anyone dropping an object has a point scored against him. At a signal, all passing stops instantly, and those holding an object have a point scored against them. The game then continues as before. A winner is determined by the lowest score after a specified playing time. The objects passed are considered to be very hot. Imagination must be used to recognize this fact. Since one's brain tells him that an object is hot and painful, he gets rid of the pain-causing element — that is by passing the object to the next person. Children acquire a fast reaction to something hot. They can understand how quickly the brain informs one of danger or other messages, and one acts accordingly to these messages.

Concept: Cold germs are spread by direct contact. One way of preventing spread of colds is by keeping away from others when one has a cold.

Activity: Circle Pass Ball

Any number of children form a single circle, facing inward. There should be a space of about three feet between players. The teacher or one child chosen to be the leader stands in the center. A ball is passed quickly from one player to another around the circle. The leader gives a signal and the child having the ball at that time has a point scored against him. This child goes to the center of the circle, and the game continues. In this game the ball represents the cold germ. The idea is to pass the ball as soon as possible so as not to be caught with the germ.

Concept: A balanced diet is good for health.

Activity: Change Circle Relay

The children make rows behind a starting line in teams of four each. About thirty feet in front of each team there are two circles drawn touching each other. In one of the circles, three ten pins or other suitable objects are placed. On a signal, the first child on each team runs up to the circles and moves the pins from the first to the second circle, then returns to the rear of his team. The second child runs up and puts the pins back in the first circle and returns in the same manner. The first team to finish is the winner. The four members of each team represent the four food groups and, if desired, can be so named. It can be pointed out that a well-balanced diet needs all four food groups; these four groups can work together to make a person healthy. The teacher can help the children to see that just as all the children on a team are needed to make it a winning team, a balanced diet is essential for good health and every type of food is important.

Concept: The circulation of the blood through the body helps the blood perform many functions.

Activity: Ball Pass

The children form a circle and pass a rubber ball around the circle to a rhythmic pattern. The first pattern could be *bounce-catch-bounce-catch;* the next could be *bounce-bounce-bounce-catch.* With two balls in play, a continuous pattern is established. The children must be alert and ready for the oncoming ball. They must also remember which pattern they are to use with the ball in play. The first child bounces the ball to a second child who catches it and bounces it on to the next child. As the second ball is put into play, the first child bounces that ball three times and, on the third bounce, sends it on to the next child. That child catches the ball and repeats the process. The balls are thought of as the blood, and the players represent the blood vessels which carry the blood to all members or parts of the body which is the entire group. When the balls make a complete circle, the children keep the balls going because blood circulates over and over. The children can understand that keeping the balls in a rhythmic pattern also helps them understand the pulse beat because they can feel it as they learn to locate the pulse in the temple, throat and wrists.

Concept: We need to guard against disease.

Activity: Hook On Tag

One child is selected to be the runner. The remaining players form groups of four. They stand one behind the other in file formation, each with arms firmly clasped around the waist of the player in front of him. The runner attempts to hook on at the end of any file where he can. File members twist and swing about trying to protect the end of their file from being caught. They must not break their arm clasps. If the runner is successful, the leader of that file becomes the new runner. The file having the most of its original members still in it at the end of a specified playing time is the winner. The runner represents a disease that the rest of the children are trying to avoid. Those who are alert, active and cooperative find that they are the ones who can avoid being tagged, and thus have a better chance to remain healthy. This activity helps the children see many ways they can avoid being exposed to germs. The main idea, of course, is to keep away from those people who might be spreading the disease.

Concept: There are many devices used as a means of safety, one of which is the traffic light.

Activity: Policeman

One child is selected to be the policeman, and sides are chosen. The sides stand equidistant from the policeman. The policeman carries a card, red on one side and green on the other. At the signal to go (green) from the policeman, each side sees how far it can get before the stop signal (red) is given. Any child who moves after the stop signal is given must go back to the original starting point. When all members of a side have passed the policeman, that side is declared the winner.

Concept: Children should know the importance of a proper diet.

Activity: Dinner's Ready

The children number off from one to five. All ones have fruit names; twos are vegetables; threes are meats; fours are milk; and fives are bread and butter. Each child is instructed to write his number and draw a picture of his category on a sheet of paper. Mother (teacher or child) beats a drum while children walk, skip, run or gallop around to the beat. When the drum stops and Mother calls, "Dinner's ready," the children must arrange themselves in circles, each containing one of each number or category of food. It is the purpose of the game to be the first food group to arrange itself. The children form themselves into balanced meals, taking one of each kind of compose a good meal. This activity is effective in teaching the components of a good meal in a short period of time.

Concept: Caution in playing with strange animals is necessary.

Activity: Dog Catcher

Half of the group of children are dog keepers and the other half are dogs. One child is designated as the dog catcher whose dog pound is marked off in a corner. The dog catcher comes out and, with his back turned, calls out, "Go!" The dogs run around teasing him, playing, barking and so on. When he turns around they may be caught and put in the pound. They keep from being caught by being on leash before he tags them. To get a leash, each dog takes his keeper's hand and stoops down. When four dogs have been caught, a new catcher is selected and keepers and dogs exchange places. In this activity, children can learn that it is important to keep dogs under control.

Concept: Various parts of the body are identified by different names.

Activity: Get Together

Half of the group are ones and the other half are twos. One player is *it*. A one becomes a partner with a two. Couples scatter over the activity area within hearing distance of *it*. *It* stands in the center and gives directions such as face to face, hands on your own thighs, hook elbows and swing, hands on your own ribs, and touch your shoulder. When *it* calls, "Get together!" all ones run for a new partner, and *it* tries to get a partner. The twos stand still and the player who fails to get a partner is *it*.

Concept: Always look up and down the street before crossing to make sure no cars are coming.

Activity: Cross the Street

The class is divided into two equal groups. An area is designated as the street and lines are drawn to indicate the width and length of the street. One group lines up on one side of the street and the other group lines up on the other side. One player on each side is selected to be a vehicle. The vehicles take their places at each end of the street rather than at the sides of the street. On a signal from the teacher, the vehicles begin to move from either end of the street. The players on the sides of the street must cross before the vehicles reach the opposite ends. All players who come close enough to the vehicles to be tagged or fail to reach the other side of the street in time have a point scored against their side. The group with the least number of points scored against it is the winner.

Concept: Fire can be harmful and destructive and we must guard against this.

Activity: Fire in the House

The players form a circle, facing the center. A ball representing fire is given to one of the players. Another ball of a different size or color, represents the house; it is given to another player approximately one-third of the way around the circle from the player with the first ball. On a signal from the teacher, the players begin to hand the fire and the house around the circle from one player to another. The idea of the game is to try to catch the house with the fire and at the same time to keep the fire from catching the house. The teacher may give a signal at certain times for the game to stop. When the game stops, a point is scored against the children who have possession of either ball. The game continues in this manner for a specified period of time.

Concept: Firemen put out fires.

Activity: Story Play (Fireman)

In story-play fashion, with the guidance of the teacher, the children act out the job of firemen from the time they leave the station until they return to the station. Children should be encouraged to suggest the activities.

Concept: We should eat certain foods to grow strong and healthy.

Activity: Fruit Basket

The players form a circle, facing the center. One player is designated as the caller and stands in the center of the circle. The players in the circle are given the names of different kinds of fruit. To start the game the caller calls out the names of two kinds of fruit. The players with those two names attempt to change places while the caller tries to tag one of them. The caller may call out, "Upset the fruit basket!" When this call is given, everyone must change to a different position. The game continues, with several children being given the opportunity to be the caller.

Concepts: Outdoor play is important to good health (exercise.) One must always watch where he is going in a running and tag game (playground safety.)

Activity: Hill Dill

Two parallel goal lines are established approximately sixty feet apart. One person is selected to be *it* and stands midway between the two goal lines. The rest of the class is divided into two equal groups with one group standing on one goal line, and the other, on the other goal line. *It* calls out, "Hill, dill, run over the hill." At this signal, the players on each of the goal lines run to the other goal line. *It* tries to tag as many as he can while they are exchanging goals. All of those tagged become helpers and the game continues in this manner until all but one have been tagged. This person is *it* for the next game.

Concepts: Erect posture is important in daily living. A strong, well-balanced framework can assume different positions. Muscles along the framework hold the body in good balance with little effort.

Activity: Attention

The class is divided into four equal groups. The members of each group stand side by side to form a line. The four lines form in such a manner that they make a square. The corners of the square should be open so that there is plenty of running space. The members of each line are numbered consecutively from left to right so that each person in a line has a different number. However, there will be four persons with the same number, one from each line. A leader calls out a number and all four persons having that number run around their own line and back to their original position. The first one back scores five points for his team, the second three points, and the third one point. The game continues in this manner for a specified period of time. All groups come to attention before each signal is given to run. When the signal is given, the others stand in a rest position.

BIBLIOGRAPHY OF RESEARCH
CONDUCTED OR DIRECTED
BY THE AUTHOR

Reading

Bobbit, Eleanor W.: *A Comparison of the Use of a Reading Readiness Workbook Approach and the Active Game Learning Medium in the Development of Selected Reading Skills and Concepts*. Ph. D. dissertation, University of Maryland, College Park, Maryland, 1972.

Humphrey, James H.: Comparison of the use of the active game learning medium with traditional procedures in the reinforcement of reading skills with fourth grade children. *Journal of Special Education*, Winter Issue, 1967.

Humphrey, James H.: Comparison of the use of active games and language workbook exercises as learning media in the development of language understandings with third grade children. *Perceptual and Motor Skills, 21*, 1965.

Humphrey, James H.: A pilot study of the use of physical education as a learning medium in the development of language arts concepts in third grade children. *Research Quarterly*, March, 1962.

Humphrey, James H., and Link, Ruth: An exploratory study of integration of physical education and reading vocabulary with selected third grade children. *Proceedings*, Research Section, American Association for Health, Physical Education and Recreation, Washington, D. C., 1959.

Humphrey, James H., and Moore, Virginia D.: Improving reading through physical education, *Education*, The Reading Issue, May, 1960.

Mathematics

Crist, Thomas: *A Comparison of the Use of the Active Game Learning Medium with Developmental-Meaningful and Drill Procedures in Developing Concepts for Telling Time at Third Grade Level*. Ph. D. dissertation, University of Maryland, College Park, Maryland, 1968.

Droter, Robert J.: *A Comparison of Active Games and Passive Games Used as Learning Media for the Development of Arithmetic Readiness Skills and Concepts With Kindergarten Children in an Attempt to Study Gross Motor Activity as a Learning Facilitator.* Master's thesis, University of Maryland, College Park, Maryland, 1972.

Humphrey, James H.: Use of the physical education learning medium in the development of certain arithmetical processes with second grade children. *Research Abstracts,* American Association for Health, Physical Education and Recreation, Washington, D. C., 1968.

Humphrey, James H.: An exploratory study of active games in learning of number concepts by first grade boys and girls. *Perceptual and Motor Skills, 23,* 1966.

Krug, Frank L.: *The Use of Physical Education Activities in the Enrichment of Learning of Certain First Grade Mathematical Concepts.* Master's thesis, University of Maryland, College Park, Maryland, 1973.

Trout, Edwin: *A Comparative Study of Selected Mathematical Concepts Developed Through Physical Education Activities Taught by the Physical Education Teacher and Traditional Techniques Taught by the Classroom Teacher.* Master's thesis, University of Maryland, College Park, Maryland, 1969.

Wright, Charles: *A Comparison of the Use of Traditional and Motor Activity Learning Media in the Development of Mathematical Concepts in Five and Six Year Old Children With an Attempt to Negate the Motivational Variable.* Master's thesis, University of Maryland, College Park, Maryland, 1969.

Science

Humphrey, James H.: The use of motor activity in the development of science concepts with mentally handicapped children. *Proceedings,* National Convention of the National Science Teachers Association, Washington, D. C., 1973.

Humphrey, James H.: The use of motor activity learning in the development of science concepts with slow learning fifth grade children. *Journal of Research in Science Teaching, 9*(3), 1972.

Humphrey, James H.: A comparison of the use of the active game learning medium and traditional media in the development of fifth grade science concepts with children with below normal intelligence quotients. *Research Abstracts,* American Association for Health, Physical Education and Recreation, Washington, D. C., 1970.

Humphrey, James H.: Developing science concepts with elementary school children through physical education. *Proceedings,* Research Section, American Association for Health, Physical Education and Recreation, Washington, D. C., 1960.

Ison, Charles: *An Experimental Study of a Comparison of the Use of Physical*

Education Activities as a Learning Medium With Traditional Teaching Procedures in the Devleopment of Selected Fifth Grade Science Concepts. Master's thesis, University of Maryland, College Park, Maryland, 1961.

Prager, Iris: *The Use of Physical Education Activities in the Reinforcement of Selected First Grade Science Concepts.* Master's thesis, University of Maryland, College Park, Maryland, 1969

INDEX